With the Compliments of

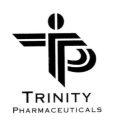

TRINITY
PHARMACEUTICALS

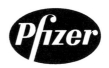

ZITHROMAX®
SUSPENSION
azithromycin

An Atlas of
PEDIATRIC INFECTIOUS DISEASES

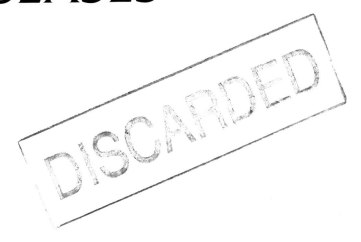

THE ENCYCLOPEDIA OF VISUAL MEDICINE SERIES

An Atlas of
PEDIATRIC INFECTIOUS DISEASES

Russell W. Steele, MD, James W. Bass, MD
and Andrew M. Margileth, MD

Professor and Vice Chairman of Pediatrics
Chief, Louisiana State University Infectious Disease Division
The Regional Medical Center for Children, New Orleans, Louisiana, USA

Senior Clinical Consultant in Pediatrics and Pediatric Infectious Diseases
Department of Pediatrics, Tripler Army Medical Center, Honolulu, Hawaii, USA

Clinical Professor of Pediatrics, Mercer University School of Medicine
Hilton Head Island, South Carolina, USA

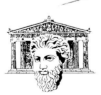

The Parthenon Publishing Group
International Publishers in Medicine, Science & Technology

NEW YORK   LONDON

Library of Congress Cataloging-in-Publication Data
Steele, Russell W., 1942–
    An atlas of pediatric infectious diseases / Russell W. Steele,
James W. Bass, and Andrew M. Margileth.
        p. cm. -- (The Encyclopedia of visual medicine series)
    Includes bibliographical references and index.
    ISBN 1-85070-914-9
        1. Infection in children--Atlases. 2. Communicable diseases in
children--Atlases. I. Bass, James W. II. Margileth, Andrew M.
III. Title. IV. Series.
        [DNLM: 1. Communicable Diseases--in infancy & childhood--
atlases. WC 17 S814a 1997]
RJ401.S84 1997
618,92'9--dc21
DNLM/DLC
for Library of Congress   97-8979
                                                                        CIP

British Library Cataloguing in Publication Data
Steele, Russell W. (Russell Wesley), 1942–
    An atlas of pediatric infectious diseases. - (The
    encyclopedia of visual medicine series)
    1. Communicable diseases in children - Atlases
    I. Title II. Bass, James W. III. Margileth, Andrew M.
    618.9'2'9

    ISBN 1-85070-914-9

Published in the USA by
The Parthenon Publishing Group Inc.
One Blue Hill Plaza
PO Box 1564, Pearl River
New York 10965, USA

Published in the UK and Europe by
The Parthenon Publishing Group Limited
Casterton Hall, Carnforth
Lancs. LA6 2LA, UK

Copyright ©1998 Parthenon Publishing Group

Printed and bound in Spain by T.G. Hostench, S.A.

Contents

Preface   7

Section I A Review of Pediatric Infectious Diseases   9

    Congenital and perinatal infections   9

    Infectious disease emergencies   10

    Maculopapular exanthematous diseases   11

    Papulovesicular exanthematous diseases   11

    Enanthems   12

    Sexually transmitted diseases   13

    Skin, soft tissue and lymph node infections   14

    Infections specific to organ systems   14

    Other infectious diseases   15

    The immunocompromised host   16

Selected bibliography   18

Section 2 Pediatric Infectious Diseases Illustrated   21

Index   99

Preface

In the care of pediatric patients, infectious diseases make up over half of diagnostic considerations. For this reason, the pediatrician or primary-care physician who is involved in the treatment of children must be particularly prepared with a basic understanding of infectious processes.

In many cases, knowledge of the disease must be applied in the clinical setting with a minimum of delay. These situations may be handled best by the physician who has access to a resource which contains a comprehensive collection of physical findings, radiographic illustrations and laboratory information pertinent to both the common as well as relatively uncommon infections. This volume, *An Atlas of Pediatric Infectious Diseases*, provides the clinician with just such a resource, aided by the use of high-quality color photographs collected by the authors over many years of clinical practice.

This atlas contains over 100 carefully selected diseases covered by more than 300 illustrations. Each topic is presented with concise yet complete diagnostic information with an emphasis on the practical aspects of management. Recent data on newly emerging infectious diseases are also highlighted.

Included among the ten chapters are infectious disease emergencies, congenital and perinatal infections, and presentations unique to the immunocompromised host. As an aid to the reader who is using the atlas to help in the diagnosis of specific patients with exanthematous diseases, additional chapters are divided according to the characteristics of the rash.

This new atlas will be an important educational and reference resource for medical students, primary-care physicians and residents who manage care for children. Furthermore, as all of these infectious diseases have been and will continue to be frequently encountered in medical practice, the information contained in this volume is unlikely to ever become out of date.

R.W. Steele
J.W. Bass
A.M. Margileth
New Orleans, LA; Honolulu, HI;
and Hilton Head Island, SC

Section 1 A Review of Pediatric Infectious Diseases

Congenital and perinatal infections

Serious infections are more common during the neonatal period than at any other time in life; this is largely a consequence of immature host defense mechanisms. During the first 28 days of life, the incidence of sepsis is reported to be as high as 8 cases per 1000 live births, with 20–25% of these having associated meningitis. Despite advances in neonatal intensive care and antibiotic therapy, mortality due to such infections remains at approximately 25%.

Neonatal sepsis can be divided into early-onset and late-onset disease, and each has distinctive features. Late-onset sepsis typically affects previously healthy infants who have been discharged from the hospital. Early clinical manifestations of neonatal sepsis are frequently non-specific and subtle, and often show overlap with symptoms of non-infectious diseases.

Well-defined perinatal factors identify which infants are at greatest risk for infection; for example, prematurity markedly increases risk. Clinical manifestations of neonatal sepsis are variable in occurrence and involve many different organ systems.

Laboratory studies may be helpful during initial clinical evaluation but, despite numerous attempts to develop more sensitive and specific rapid laboratory tests for infection, the white blood cell (WBC) count and differential remain the most frequently used screening studies. Neutropenia, especially an absolute neutrophil count $<1800/mm^3$ or an immature neutrophil-to-total neutrophil ratio of >0.15 during the first 24 h of life are strongly suggestive of infection. Leukocytosis, defined as a WBC count $>25\,000/mm^3$, may also be the result of infection, but is more often associated with non-infectious causes.

Other hematological findings in neonatal infection include thrombocytopenia, WBC vacuolization and toxic granulations. Rapid antigen-detection tests, such as latex-particle agglutination or countercurrent immunoelectrophoresis, offer supportive evidence for specific bacterial etiologies, but false-positive results have limited their usefulness. Numerous other adjunctive tests, including C-reactive protein and erythrocyte sedimentation rate (ESR) tests, have been used to screen for sepsis, but none have been widely accepted.

Cultures of blood and cerebrospinal fluid (CSF) should be obtained from all neonates with suspected sepsis, although clinical judgment should be exercised to determine the safety of lumbar puncture in infants at risk for respiratory compromise or preterm infants at risk for intraventricular hemorrhage. Tracheal aspirate cultures, when available, are useful in infants with respiratory symptoms, although endotracheal tube colonization is inevitable with prolonged intubation. Urine culture is of low yield in the evaluation of early-onset infection, but is useful in late-onset infection. Urine for culture should be obtained by suprapubic aspiration of the bladder when possible. Gastric aspirate and skin cultures may reflect bacterial colonization at birth, but do not always correlate with systemic infection. Chest radiography is indicated in infants with respiratory distress as a screen for both pneumonia and non-infectious causes.

Normal values for CSF in neonates differ from those in older infants. Cerebrospinal fluid WBC counts as high as $30/mm^3$, protein values of 170 mg/dl and glucose values as low as 24 mg/dl are normal during the neonatal period.

Congenital infections with non-bacterial pathogens also result in significant morbidity and mortality. TORCH is the acronym for what were once the more common pathogens involved in congenital infections: *Toxoplasma* species, rubella virus, cytomegalovirus (CMV) and herpes simplex virus.

Clinical manifestations of intrauterine infections are variable and there is considerable overlap among the different pathogens. Findings which should arouse suspicion for congenital disease include intrauterine growth retardation, microcephaly, hepatosplenomegaly, anemia and thrombocytopenia. It should be noted, however, that most cases of intrauterine growth retardation and microcephaly are not caused by infection.

Infectious disease emergencies

Some infectious disease presentations should be diagnosed and treated rapidly to prevent mortality and provide the optimal prognosis. In many cases, therapy must be instituted before a diagnosis can be confirmed. These are true emergencies and, fortunately, only a few such entities are commonly encountered in pediatric patients.

Sepsis and meningitis are the two most commonly seen emergencies. In most cases, only one or two laboratory specimens need to be obtained before treatment is begun. In other instances, only supportive therapy is warranted, either because specific treatment is not yet available or because eradication of the invading pathogen is not necessary. Such entities include viral encephalitis (other than herpes simplex virus or varicella–zoster virus), viral myocarditis, Reye's syndrome, Guillain–Barré syndrome, infant botulism and rabies.

The clinician's assessment of toxicity remains the most sensitive test for determining which children have early, but potentially severe, bacterial infections. Such assessment has been carefully defined and quantitated using criteria referred to as the Yale Observation Scale. There are eight categories in this scoring system:

(1) Feeding history
(2) Reaction to the environment
(3) Irritability
(4) Consolability
(5) Absence of social smile
(6) Quality of the cry
(7) Color
(8) Hydration.

A judgment that a child fulfills criteria for toxicity has an impact on decisions for the diagnostic workup, such as cultures, measurement of, for example, acute phase reactants, hospitalization and empirical antimicrobial therapy.

Prior to 1990, the most common cause of life-threatening and fatal bacterial infections in children was *Haemophilus influenzae* type b (Hib). However, now that conjugate Hib vaccines are routinely administered to young children, this pathogen is rarely encountered in pediatric practice. At present, *Streptococcus pneumoniae* and *Neisseria meningitidis* are the two bacterial organisms causing most cases of bacteremia which progress to shock with multi-organ failure or produce focal infection, such as meningitis, pneumonia and purulent pericarditis. Other pathogens which have reemerged as common etiologies of severe infection are group A beta-hemolytic streptococci and *Staphylococcus aureus*.

Many of the bacterial infections included in Section 2 will progress to septic shock if not treated early and aggressively. Selection of empirical antibiotic therapy depends on the clinical setting, early clues for etiological diagnosis and on a thorough knowledge of microbial susceptibility patterns.

Most infectious disease emergencies should be managed in a well-equipped intensive care unit, at least during the acute phase of illness. By definition, progression of disease may require endotracheal intubation or other specialized support procedures. For this reason, transport to referral medical centers should be considered if local facilities do not include intensive-care capabilities.

Maculopapular exanthematous diseases

The rashes of the exanthematous diseases of childhood can be broadly separated into those which are primarily erythematous maculopapular and those which are papulovesicular (see below). These classifications represent the starting point used by clinicians in formulating a differential diagnosis during initial examination and management. Additional data for diagnosis are the prodrome, other diagnostic signs and laboratory tests.

The following are the most common and most often misdiagnosed diseases associated with maculopapular rashes:

Drug eruptions
Enteroviral infections
Epstein–Barr virus infections
Erythema infectiosum
Erythema multiforme minor
Kawasaki disease
Measles
Roseola
Rubella
Scarlet fever
Staphylococcal scalded skin syndrome.

Macular rashes which mimic measles (morbilli) are often referred to as morbilliform eruptions. Macules are otherwise defined as color changes of the skin that are flat (not palpable) whereas papules are raised with distinct borders measuring 1 cm or less. Many exanthems exhibit a combination of macules and papules, and are thus referred to as maculopapular eruptions.

Viruses induce skin rashes either by direct invasion of the skin, where they replicate within keratinocytes (epidermotropic), or by indirectly producing skin reactivity by mechanisms that remain poorly defined. Lesions are usually generalized. However, the majority have a photodistribution as exposure to the sun enhances the intensity of these rashes.

Maculopapular eruptions are the most common form of viral-induced exanthems and therefore constitute the most frequent differential diagnosis. Many maculopapular eruptions are of non-infectious etiology, most commonly drug induction. Because of their frequent use, antibiotics are often incriminated. Reactive erythema due to trauma or sensitivity to sunlight may also mimic viral exanthems.

Papulovesicular exanthematous diseases

Papules and vesicles are sharply circumscribed elevated lesions < 1 cm in diameter. Vesicles contain non-purulent fluid. Often, these lesions evolve from papules to vesicles which rupture to produce ulcerated craters, scales or crusts. Secondary colonization with common skin flora, particularly *S. aureus* and group A streptococci, may produce impetigo, cellulitis or subcutaneous abscesses.

Papulovesicular eruptions often present with many stages of development and a combination of secondary features. Non-infectious etiologies are numerous. Examples of lesions that are papular, but non-vesicular, are nevi and lichen planus. The most common entities that vesiculate include dyshydrosis and contact dermatitis.

Many viral and bacterial pathogens produce papular and/or vesicular exanthems. One of these, smallpox or variola, was successfully eradicated worldwide and is now of historical interest only.

The most common and often misdiagnosed diseases characterized by papulovesicular eruptions are:

> Coxsackie virus infections
> Eczema herpeticum
> Gianotti–Crosti syndrome
> Herpetic whitlow
> Impetigo
> Molluscum contagiosum
> Papular urticaria
> Varicella–zoster.

Clinical features which help to differentiate infections should be particularly noted. These include the distribution of the rash, associated enanthems, presence of fever or other constitutional symptoms and unique associated findings.

Enanthems

Examination of the oral cavity not only provides information on patients whose primary complaint relates to the mouth or throat, but may also yield important diagnostic clues to systemic disease. The state of hydration may be assessed by the amount of moisture on mucous membranes; the pallor of anemia may be noted, and cyanosis of the lips is evidence of congenital heart disease. Malodorous breath is associated with tissue breakdown from infection, particularly anaerobes as with Vincent's angina, but may also provide the first indication of liver disease or diabetes mellitus.

Lesions in the oral cavity may be structural defects, inflammatory, neoplastic or post-traumatic as well as of infectious etiology. In addition, there are some non-infectious etiologies which have appearances similar to the enanthems (see Section 2).

One of the most common structural abnormalities is the mucocele. These are lesions at the site of minor salivary glands. Epstein pearls are white nodular cystic structures located along the alveolar ridge in young infants, and dermoid cysts may appear along the anterior floor of the mouth. A torus palatinus is a bony defect of the hard palate seen in 20% of adolescents, and a fibrosing mucocele is a similar developmental abnormality of the mucous membrane covering the palate.

The most common inflammatory disorder is erythema multiforme of the mouth, which is often associated with a skin rash and conjunctivitis. The severe form is called Stevens–Johnson syndrome. Other common inflammatory lesions include gingival hyperplasia and lichen planus.

Most important among the differentials are malignant neoplasms, but these are generally larger masses. Unlike oral tumors in adults, the lesions in children are usually sarcomas, with rhabdomyosarcoma predominating. With tissue breakdown, these may be confused with abscesses, cellulitis or other infectious lesions.

Trauma to the oral mucosa and injuries from sharp objects such as pencils or popsicle sticks are most likely to imitate enanthems associated with infectious diseases. A careful history for trauma should thus be obtained if lesions are not completely characteristic of other etiologies.

Sexually transmitted diseases

Sexually transmitted diseases (STDs) can be broadly divided into those characterized by genital ulcers with or without inguinal adenopathy, infections of epithelial surfaces, and specific well-defined syndromes. Genital ulcers are most commonly associated with herpes simplex, syphilis or, less commonly, chancroid, and may be differentiated by the presence or absence of pain. Syphilis is usually painless whereas herpes and chancroid are painful.

Depending on the specific findings and other features such as adenopathy [syphilis, lymphogranuloma venereum (LGV) and chancroid], evaluation of genital ulcers should include the following: dark-field examination or direct immunofluorescence tests for *Treponema pallidum*; serological tests for syphilis; culture, Tzanck tests or fluorescence stains for herpes simplex virus (HSV); and culture for *Haemophilus ducreyi*.

The appearances of the skin lesions are often diagnostic. Genital warts (papillomavirus), ecchymoses of the arthritis–dermatitis syndrome (*N. gonorrhoeae*) and the multiple painful ulcers of HSV are readily recognizable.

STDs may also be classified according to their specific pathogens, but this is less practical than an etiological diagnosis on the basis of clinical presentations. An example is urethritis, which may be the result of bacteria, viruses or even protozoa.

The classical STD triad of syphilis, gonorrhea and chancroid now accounts for only a fraction of the currently recognized pathogens. Indeed, they have been largely replaced by *Chlamydia trachomatis*, hepatitis B and human immunodeficiency virus (HIV) as major diseases.

With the increasing prevalence of STDs, physicians have emphasized methods of prevention, particularly among adolescents, and have become more aware of the variable presentations, the potential seriousness of the sequelae for children born to infected mothers and the implications of the diagnosis of an acquired STD in a prepubescent child in terms of child abuse. All of these are issues with which the clinicians who treat children should be familiar.

Because multiple STDs frequently coexist in the same patient, the detection of one disease requires examination for others, regardless of the presenting symptoms. Careful physical examination, including the oropharynx, rectum, genitalia and skin, should be performed. Laboratory studies include urinalysis, selected serological tests based on clinical findings, Gram stains of cervical or urethral discharge, wet mounts of vaginal secretions, diagnostic tests for *C. trachomatis* on cervical (vaginal in prepubertal girls) or urethral specimens, and cultures of the oropharynx, rectum and cervix or penile urethra for *N. gonorrhoeae*. The detection of HIV infection often alters the management of STDs, particularly syphilis, which would then require higher dosages of penicillin and a longer duration of therapy.

It is frequently forgotten that infection in a neonate or young infant with a pathogen which is transmitted through sexual contact warrants evaluation and treatment of the mother as well as her sexual contacts. Examples include gonococcal ophthalmia, chlamydial conjunctivitis and pneumonia, congenital syphilis and HIV. Mothers with these infections are frequently asymptomatic.

STDs in children may have been acquired by sexual contact. Recent studies suggest that approximately 20% of children and adolescents have been sexually abused by the age of 21 years. Sexual abuse is generally perpetrated by someone known to the child and frequently continues over a prolonged period of time. If the sexual-abuse event occurred more than 72 h before evaluation, specimens should be collected for evaluation of the common STDs. If the abuse was more recent, then the appropriate forensic specimens should be collected. However, the collection of specimens for evaluation of STDs may be delayed.

Antimicrobial treatment should be considered if:

(1) The alleged perpetrator was known to be infected with an STD;
(2) More than one assailant was involved;
(3) The patient is unlikely to return for follow-up;
(4) The patient or parents are anxious regarding the possibility of acquiring an STD.

When evaluating a child for possible sexual abuse, appropriate tests for gonorrhea, chlamydial infection, HIV and syphilis (as well as for other infections in selected circumstances) should be obtained. Evaluating physicians should identify those patients suspected of being victims of sexual abuse who thus warrant laboratory evaluation for an STD. Some experts advise culturing all children examined for sexual abuse for *C. trachomatis* and *N. gonorrhoeae* as many abused children do not disclose the extent of their abuse, and infection with these agents may be asymptomatic.

Skin, soft tissue and lymph node infections

Infectious diseases which affect the skin and skin structures allow ready application of diagnostic skills, and access to microscopic evaluation and culture of the offending pathogen. In addition, there are some diseases which are associated with skin lesions as a result of toxin production, immune complex formation or delayed hypersensitivity reactions to antigens from responsible microbes.

Soft-tissue infections may be the result of direct inoculation of the skin, bacteremia and hematogenous spread from another site, lymphogenous proliferation of pathogens or extension from contiguous disease. Microorganisms may produce abscesses, affect vascular structures causing visible changes or alter extravascular structures of the dermis.

Many factors need to be borne in mind when making early clinical diagnoses. Characteristics of the skin lesions are the first consideration. Vesicular, bullous, petechial, pustular, ulcerated or nodular lesions each suggest a specific etiology in a differential diagnosis. The location of the lesions separates many similar entities; chronic submandibular adenopathy is more indicative of atypical mycobacterial disease whereas similar lymphatic involvement in the axillae is suggestive of cat-scratch disease.

When a specific etiology is strongly suspected on clinical grounds alone and the patient is asymptomatic or only mildly ill, an empirical course of therapy without further diagnostic testing is appropriate. This significantly reduces the cost of medical care. Most of the infections included in this atlas (see Section 2) fall into this category when pathogens are predictable. Laboratory confirmation may only be necessary to identify unusual antimicrobial susceptibility patterns or to separate a few possibilities within a differential diagnosis.

Infections specific to organ systems

Young children often develop infection with common colonizing bacteria because they lack antibody to these organisms and because their immune responses are decreased compared with those of adults. Important potential pathogens include *Streptococcus pneumoniae*, *H. influenzae*, *N. meningi-*

tidis, *S. aureus* and group A beta-hemolytic streptococci. These five groups predominate in children during the preschool years following infancy, and are responsible for bacteremia, sepsis and serious focal infections, such as cellulitis, pericarditis, osteomyelitis, pneumonia and meningitis.

With any febrile illness, it is important that the clinician look for clues that may differentiate the usual self-limited viral infections from bacterial disease of greater consequence. This is generally achieved by an assessment of 'toxicity', as the child with early bacterial infection is more likely to manifest clinical changes indicative of infection of greater consequence.

There are eight general categories for the assessment of toxicity:

(1) Feeding history

(2) State of hydration

(3) Reaction to the environment

(4) Irritability

(5) Consolability

(6) Absence of a social smile

(7) Quality of the cry

(8) Color changes (such as pallor and cyanosis).

The sensitivity of this clinical assessment is approximately 75% for determining serious illness, which is higher than that of any laboratory test currently available.

The site of infection may not cause obvious focal signs and symptoms; examples are urinary tract infection, brain abscesses and osteomyelitis. Therefore, for any patient with a suspected bacterial illness, blood cultures should be obtained. However, even in cases with an obvious focus, blood cultures may be positive whereas the local site may prove negative on culture.

Early antibiotic therapy for children with a high fever, but no identifiable focus of infection, remains highly controversial. Although some studies have shown benefit with early empirical therapy, the increasing antibiotic resistance of organisms such as *S. pneumoniae* to the most commonly used agents for treatment argue against their routine use in all children considered at risk for occult bacteremia. It would probably be best for the physician to individualize cases by examining all young children carefully for toxicity and for early signs of focal disease.

Other infectious diseases

Non-bacterial pathogens account for a significant percentage of infections in children. These are predominantly viruses, which comprise the etiology of most upper and lower respiratory tract infections, and most self-limited febrile illnesses.

Although fungal diseases constitute a small percentage of disease, they may be life-threatening particularly if diagnosis is delayed. *Pneumocystis carinii*, now classified as a fungus, is the predominant cause of life-threatening pneumonia in children with HIV infection, and is usually treated with trimethoprim-sulfamethoxazole. Other mycoses are treated with amphotericin B, imidazoles (clotrimazole, miconazole and ketoconazole) or triazoles (fluconazole and itraconazole).

Rickettsiae are unique bacterial pathogens and are treated with tetracyclines or chloramphenicol. Antimicrobial therapy for these pathogens is therefore very different from that required for most bacterial pathogens, for which the cephalosporins or penicillins are usually employed. However, none of the rickettsiae are susceptible to these classes of antibiotics.

Parasitic diseases have virtually disappeared in the developed countries as a result of concentrated efforts to improve sanitary conditions. Malaria and intestinal nematodes, previously common in all regions, are now only encountered in patients who have traveled to tropical developing countries. Only pinworm (enterobiasis) and giardiasis are seen with any frequency in pediatric practices, with occasional cases of ascariasis, amebiasis, strongyloidiasis, toxocariasis, hookworm and whipworm (trichuriasis) requiring management.

The immunocompromised host

Reduced host defense responses may be the result of congenital abnormalities (primary immunodeficiency) or may be secondary to certain disease processes, such as cancer and autoimmune disorders, wherein host responses are worsened by the immunosuppressive chemotherapy.

Initial clinical manifestations are often infections due to pathogens that are rarely seen in the immune-competent host or severe disease caused by relatively non-virulent microbial agents. The type of pathogen (viral, fungal, extracellular bacteria or intracellular bacteria) often suggests the compartment of immune function – cellular, humoral or phagocytic – that is most affected.

It is difficult to determine the incidence of primary immunodeficiency syndromes as many of the more severe forms may result in early infant death before a diagnosis can be made. In one recent study, it was estimated that one of every 50 deaths in children was a result of immune dysfunction.

In actual clinical practice, however, the more severe defects are only occasionally encountered by primary-care physicians. It is the more common deficiencies, such as transient hypogammaglobulinemia of infancy and selective IgA deficiency, that are familiar to most clinicians. Other syndromes more likely to be encountered include common variable hypogammaglobulinemia, chronic mucocutaneous candidiasis, cyclic neutropenia, Bruton's X-linked hypogammaglobulinemia, severe combined immune deficiency, Wiskott–Aldrich syndrome and complement deficiencies. Only selected infectious disease aspects of these syndromes are included in this atlas (see Section 2).

The importance of measuring immune competence is more greatly appreciated as defects in immunity become increasingly implicated in disease processes. More importantly, early recognition of immune deficiency is critical for the successful treatment of patients, both in terms of managing the primary disease and anticipating secondary complications.

Initial presentations may be subtle. On retrospective reviewing of the clinical histories of patients with documented immunodeficiency, it becomes apparent that the first encounter with a physician is for treatment of an apparently trivial illness such as pneumonia, a focal bacterial infection, a prolonged viral illness or perhaps simply oral thrush.

All physicians should, as part of patient management, consider etiology and ask why this particular patient should have developed this particular disease. If the reason for the predisposition is apparent (it is the patient's first encounter with influenza virus resulting in pneumonia), then a satisfactory answer is available. If an explanation is not apparent, (the patient has P. carinii pneumonia), then the physician should consider a thorough screen of immune function in this patient.

Most of these deficiencies present during infancy or early childhood; the most notable exceptions are common variable hypogammaglobulinemia, cyclic neutropenia and complement deficiencies, all of which may not become clinically apparent until later in life.

Deficiencies of the later components of complement (C5–8) are not seen until adolescence or early adulthood, with the presentation of recurrent meningococcal and gonococcal disease.

Secondary suppression of immunological function with resultant increased susceptibility to infection may occur as a result of a number of primary diseases. Oncology patients and others receiving immunosuppressive therapy have been evaluated to stage their susceptibility to infectious diseases in a manner similar to staging the prognosis in cancer. These are the patients who later may come to demonstrate disseminated varicella–zoster, *P. carinii* pneumonia, disseminated herpes simplex or bacterial sepsis.

Antimicrobial prophylaxis and early treatment are an important aspect of the management of such patients. Some will also benefit from such immuno-therapeutic approaches as intravenous immunoglobulin or granulocyte colony-stimulating factor as part of their overall care. This circumstance is more common in adults than in children because of the higher incidence of malignancy and greater use of immunosuppressive chemotherapy for a variety of diseases. The acquired immunodeficiency syndrome (AIDS) is the most common predisposing immunodeficiency in children.

Over 2% of all hospitalized children demonstrate secondary defects in host resistance. Recognition and treatment of these host defense abnormalities have therefore become an important aspect of hospital practice. Secondary deficiency is, in fact, much more common than primary immunological disorder even in infants and children, and can be adequately managed by primary-care physicians with consultative support.

Selected bibliography

Congenital and perinatal infections

Steele RW. *The Clinical Handbook of Pediatric Infectious Disease.* Carnforth: Parthenon Publishing, 1994:49–66

Henderson JL, Weiner CP. Congenital infection. *Curr Opin Obstet Gynecol* 1995;2:130–4

Epps RE, Pittelkow MR, Su WP. TORCH syndrome. *Semin Dermatol* 1995;14:179–86

Steele RW. Prevention of group B streptococcal infection in pregnant women and neonates. *Infect Med* 1996;13:382–96

Infectious disease emergencies

Harper MB. Pediatric infectious disease emergencies. *Curr Opin Pediatr* 1995;7:302–8

Foltin GL. Critical issues in urban emergency medical services for children. *Pediatrics* 1995;96:174–9

Bisno AL, Stevens DL. Streptococcal infections of skin and soft tissues. *N Engl J Med* 1996;334:240–5

Bass JW, Steele RW, Wiebe RA. Acute epiglottitis, a surgical emergency. *JAMA* 1974;229:761–5

Bass JW, Steele RW, Wittler RR, *et al.* Antimicrobial treatment of occult bacteremia: A multicenter cooperative study. *Pediatr Infect Dis J* 1993;12:466–73

Maculopapular exanthematous diseases

Hurwitz S. *Clinical Pediatric Dermatology.* Philadelphia: WB Saunders Co, 1993

Frieden IJ. Childhood exanthems. *Curr Opin Pediatr* 1995;7:411–4

Krugman S, Katz SL, Gershon AA, *et al. Infectious Diseases of Children.* St Louis: Mosby Year Book, 1992

Hartley AH, Rasmussen JE. Infectious exanthems. *Pediatr Rev* 1988;9:321–6

Newburger JW, Takahashi M, Beiser AS, *et al.* A single intravenous infusion of gamma globulin as compared with four infusions in the treatment of acute Kawasaki syndrome. *N Engl J Med* 1991;324:1633–9

Papulovesicular exanthematous diseases

Rudolph AM, Hoffman JIE, Rudolph CD. *Rudolph's Pediatrics.* 20th edn. Stamford, CT: Appleton & Lange, 1996:499–689

American Academy of Pediatrics Committee on Infectious Diseases. Recommendations for the use of live attenuated varicella vaccine. *Pediatrics* 1995;95:791–6

Tieb A, Plantin P, DuPasquier P. Gianotti–Crosti

syndrome: A study of 26 cases. *Br J Dermatol* 1986;115:49–59

Prasad SM. Molluscum contagiosum. *Pediatr Rev* 1996;17:118–9

Shriner DL, Schwartz RA, Janniger CK. Impetigo. *Cutis* 1995;56:30–2

Enanthems

Behrman RE. *Nelson Textbook of Pediatrics.* Philadelphia: WB Saunders Co, 1992:823–31

Rogers RS. Recurrent aphthous stomatitis clinical characteristics and evidence for an immunopathogenesis. *J Invest Dermatol* 1977;69:499–509

Sexually transmitted diseases

Holmes KK, Mardh P, Sparling PF, *et al. Sexually Transmitted Diseases.* New York: McGraw–Hill, Inc, 1990

American Academy of Pediatrics (AAP). *Summaries of Infectious Diseases. 1994 Red Book.* 23rd edn. Elk Grove Village, IL: AAP, 1994:115–520

CDC. 1993 Sexually transmitted diseases treatment guidelines. *MMWR* 1993;44:1–102

Stone KM. Human papillomavirus infection and genital warts: Update on epidemiology and treatment. *Clin Infect Dis* 1995;20:S91–7

Horner TM, Guyer MJ, Kalter NM. Clinical expertise and the assessment of child sexual abuse. *J Am Acad Child Adolesc Psychiatr* 1993;32:925–31

Skin, soft tissue and lymph node infections

Minnick KE, Dillon PW. Pediatric soft tissue infections. *Semin Pediatr Surg* 1995;4:228–33

Goldstein EJC. Bite wounds and infection. *Clin Infect Dis* 1992;14:633–40

Margileth AM, Hayden GB. Cat-scratch disease: From feline affection to human infection. *N Engl J Med* 1993;329:53–4

Steele RW, Schexnayder RE, Glasier CM. Lymphadenitis in infants and children: Recognizing the unusual causes. *Infect Med* 1992;9:41–8

Jacobs RF, Narain JP. Tularemia in children. *Pediatr Infect Dis J* 1983;2:487–91

Infections specific to organ systems

Saez-Llorens XJ, Umana MA, Odio CM, *et al.* Brain abscess in infants and children. *Pediatr Infect Dis J* 1989;8:449–58

Whitley RJ. Viral encephalitis. *N Engl J Med* 1990; 323:242–50

Tan TQ, Seilheimer DK, Kaplan SL. Pediatric lung abscess: Clinical management and outcome. *Pediatr Infect Dis J* 1995;14:51–5

Cantwell MF, Snider DE, Cauthen GM, *et al.* Epidemiology of tuberculosis in the United States, 1985 through 1992. *JAMA* 1994;272:535–9

Gold R. Diagnosis of osteomyelitis. *Pediatr Rev* 1991;12:292–7

Other infectious diseases

Gaasch WH. Guidelines for the diagnosis of rheumatic fever: Jones criteria, 1992 update. *JAMA* 1992;268:2069–73

Steele RW. Diagnosis and management of rickettsial diseases. *Infect Med* 1989;6:97–102

Liu L, Weller PF. Antiparasitic drugs. *N Engl J Med* 1996;334:1178–84

Pearson RD, Sousa AQ. Clinical spectrum of leishmaniasis. *Clin Infect Dis* 1996;22:1–13

Sinnott JT, Oehler RL, Baran DA, *et al.* Relapsing fever. *Infect Med* 1992;9:18–24

The immunocompromised host

Kaplan JE, Masur H, Holmes KK. Prevention of opportunistic infections in persons infected with human immunodeficiency virus. *Clin Infect Dis* 1995; 21:S1–141

Forrest CB, Forehand JR, Axtell RA, *et al.* Clinical features and current management of chronic granulomatous disease. *Hematol Oncol Clin North Am* 1988;2:253–66

Stiehm ER. New and old immunodeficiencies. *Pediatr Res* 1992;33:S2–8

Lerner PI. Nocardiosis. *Clin Infect Dis* 1996;22: 891–905

Choo PW, Donahue JG, Manson JE, *et al.* The epidemiology of varicella and its complications. *J Infect Dis* 1995;172:706–12

Section 2 Pediatric Infectious Diseases Illustrated

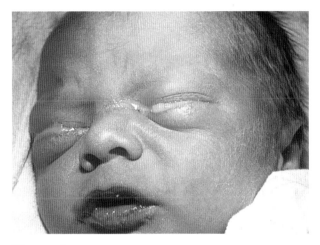

Figure 1

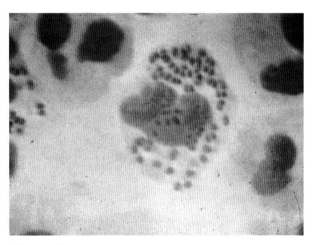

Figure 2

Congenital and perinatal infections

Conjunctivitis

The causes of conjunctivitis are largely age-dependent in neonates and young infants, and include sensitivity to topical chemicals and environmental allergens as well as viral and bacterial pathogens. The most common etiology during the first 3 days of life is the prophylactic application of silver nitrate (Figure 1) and, to a lesser extent, erythromycin or tetracycline; no treatment is necessary.

From 3 days to 3 weeks of life, *Neisseria gonorrhoeae* produces ophthalmia neonatorum, which is best confirmed by Gram-staining (Figure 2) and culture of a conjunctival scraping. *Chlamydia trachomatis* produces conjunctivitis (inclusion blennorrhea) at 3–20 weeks of age. Identification can be made by Giemsa-staining of a conjunctival scraping to reveal

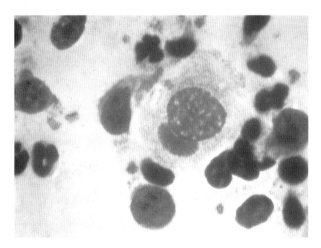

Figure 3

paranuclear elementary bodies within the epithelial cells (Figure 3). However, this method has only a 30% sensitivity compared with culture or direct fluorescent staining. Other causes of bacterial con-

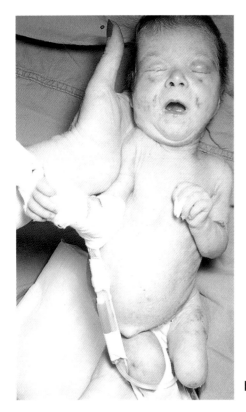

Figure 4

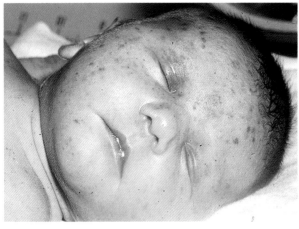

Figure 5

junctivitis after day 2 of life are *Staphylococcus aureus*, streptococci and coliforms.

Cytomegalovirus

Cytomegalovirus (CMV) may be vertically transmitted to the fetus during primary or recurrent maternal infection, but only 4% of infected infants are symptomatic at birth. These infants have a mortality rate of 25% and almost all survivors have long-term morbidity. Of the 96% of infected infants who

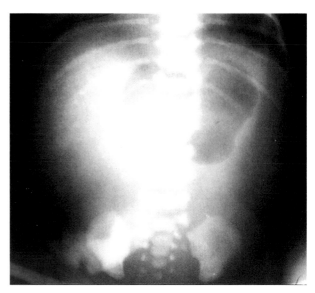

Figure 6

are asymptomatic at birth, up to 15% will develop significant late neurological sequelae, with sensorineural hearing loss being the most common. Diagnosis is confirmed by recovery of CMV from the urine or a target organ.

This 8-week-old infant (Figure 4), who was small for gestational age, had congenital CMV infection and presented with the classical features of purpura, hepatosplenomegaly, microcephaly, severe anemia, thrombocytopenia and leukocytosis. Chest X-ray revealed interstitial infiltrates. CMV was cultured from the urine. Failure to thrive, respiratory distress, recurrent epistaxis and ascites persisted; death ensued at 9 weeks of age.

Other manifestations of congenital infection are jaundice (Figure 5), chorioretinitis and intracerebral, usually periventricular, calcifications. Another rare but specific radiological finding is intrahepatic calcifications (Figure 6).

Group B streptococcal cellulitis–adenitis in infants

A unique presentation of infection due to group B streptococcus (GBS) in pediatric patients <3 months of age (Figure 7) was originally termed 'facial or submandibular cellulitis in young infants'. Illness begins with fever, irritability and decreased

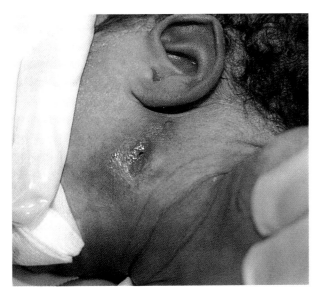

Figure 7

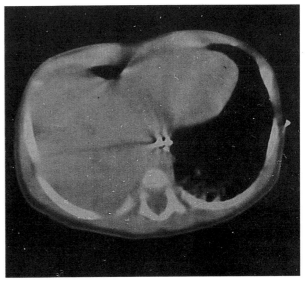

Figure 9

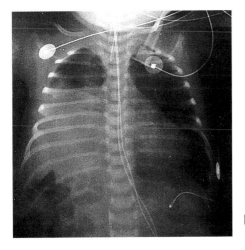

Figure 8

feeding, rapidly followed by swelling and erythema in the facial, submandibular or inguinal region. Local adenitis is a prominent feature and often provides a source of culture and identification of GBS.

Similar infection caused by *Staphylococcus aureus* rarely causes nodes to suppurate or to require surgical drainage. Two other contrasting features are that almost all patients with GBS disease are bacteremic, and the majority develop ipsilateral otitis media. The age of these pediatric patients (< 3 months old) should also differentiate them from those with other etiologies.

The mean age of onset is 5 weeks. There is a prevalence of serotype III strains, and recovery of the

same organism from the maternal vaginal and / or rectal cultures is frequent, all of which serve to support cellulitis-adenitis as another manifestation of late-onset GBS disease transmitted by the mother. Management should therefore include a sepsis work-up with examination of the cerebrospinal fluid (CSF), and careful evaluation of bones and joints to rule out other foci of infection.

Group B streptococci are the leading cause of early-onset sepsis in neonates and most commonly present as severe pneumonia during the first 48 h of life. Pulmonary infection may occasionally produce a diaphragmatic hernia, as seen in this 10-day-old neonate (Figure 8). Computed tomography (CT) of the chest confirmed protrusion of the liver through a defect in the right diaphragm (Figure 9). Severe pneumonia at 2 h of life required intubation and antimicrobial therapy. Multiple blood cultures were positive for GBS. The hernia was not present prior to day 10 of life.

Herpes simplex viruses (HSV)

Herpes simplex virus types 1 (15%) and 2 (85%) cause maternal herpes genitalis and may result in perinatal infection. Neonatal disease presents during the first 42 days of life as a rapidly evolving disease with clinical symptoms similar to those of bacterial sepsis. Most infected infants are born to

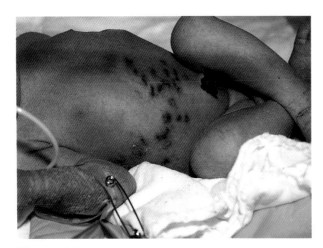

Figure 10

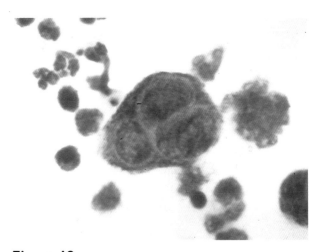

Figure 12

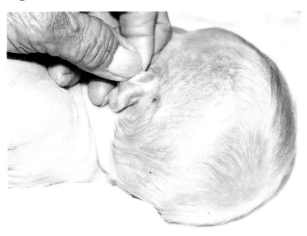

Figure 11

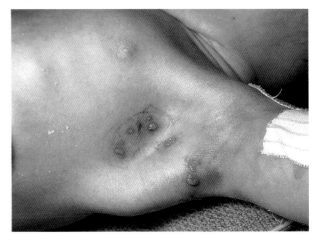

Figure 13

mothers who are asymptomatic, but who shed the virus from a reactivated genital infection at the time of delivery.

Neonatal disease may be categorized into three classifications: localized infection of the skin (Figure 10), eyes or mouth; central nervous system (CNS) infection with or without skin, eye or mouth involvement; and disseminated infection. Mortality is highest for infants with disseminated disease and morbidity is high for infants with disseminated or CNS infection.

Diagnosis can be confirmed by culture of the virus from skin vesicles, mucosal lesions, blood or CSF. Skin lesions may be subtle; this neonate (Figure 11) had a single vesicle behind the ear. Cytological examination with fluorescence, or a Tzanck preparation using Wright- or Giemsa-staining of lesion scrapings, may also be helpful in the diagnosis by identifying multinucleated giant cells (Figure 12).

This 12-day-old infant (Figure 13) had encephalitis diagnosed at age 6 days. Herpes simples virus type 2 was recovered from vesicles in the axilla. The infant developed profound mental retardation and death occurred 3 months later. No antimicrobial therapy was given.

Another presentation is bronchopneumonia (Figure 14), as in this severely ill neonate who had no skin manifestations or other organ involvement.

Herpes may occasionally manifest as a true congenital infection following infection *in utero* during the first or second trimester of pregnancy, and cause growth retardation and deep dermal scars (Figures 15 and 16).

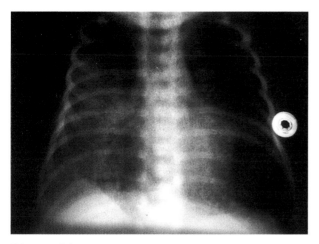

Figure 14

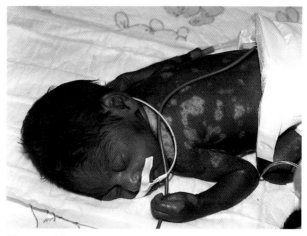

Figure 16

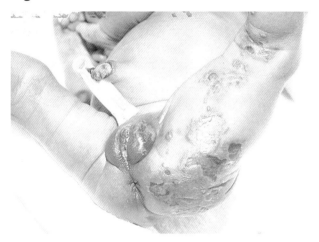

Figure 15

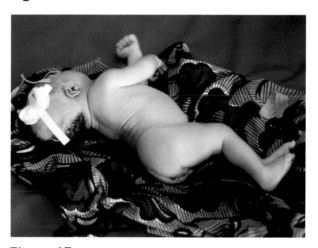

Figure 17

Neonatal tetanus

This neonate developed opisthotonus 4 days after delivery (Figure 17). His umbilical cord had been cut by a midwife using an unsterilized instrument. The causative organism is *Clostridium tetani*, present in the environment primarily in the form of spores.

Once introduced into a wound, however, the spores convert to the vegetative form, producing the potent toxin tetanospasmin which affects the CNS and causing a variety of neurological and systemic manifestations, including seizures, and spasm of laryngeal and respiratory musculature, with airway obstruction, fever, tachycardia, hypertension, cardiac arrhythmias and urinary retention.

The most commonly affected cranial nerves are III, IV, VII, IX, X and XI. The incubation period is 3 days to 3 weeks. Neonates usually present during the first week of life with difficulty in sucking, dysphagia, excessive crying, spasms and opisthotonus.

Mortality for neonatal tetanus is 80–90%. The condition is common in countries where women do not receive tetanus immunization, and accounts for an estimated 600 000 deaths / year. Recovery from tetanus does not confer immunity, so active immunization still needs to be offered.

Omphalitis

This is infection of the umbilical stump, usually caused by *Staphylococcus aureus*, group A beta-hemolytic or group B streptococci, or Gram-negative enteric bacilli, and may extend into the umbilical and portal veins to produce bacteremia and sepsis. Omphalitis is a true medical emergency.

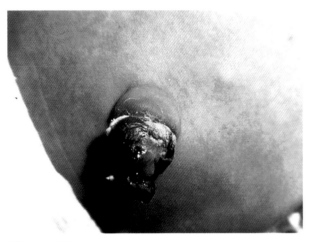

Figure 18

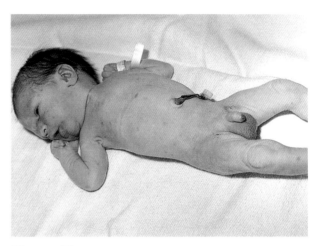

Figure 19

Infection of the umbilical cord without extension (funisitis) presents at birth in association with chorioamnionitis whereas omphalitis tends to develop after 3–10 days. This severely ill 7-day-old infant (Figure 18) has omphalitis and bacteremia due to *S. aureus*.

Rubella

Transplacentally acquired during the course of primary maternal disease, rubella virus infection during fetal development may result in growth retardation, heart defects, hepatosplenomegaly, thrombocytopenia, cataracts, glaucoma and deafness. The incidence and severity of malformations are increased if infection occurs early in gestation.

Diagnosis can be made by virus isolation or by testing for IgM antibody to rubella. Treatment is supportive and infected infants require isolation as virus excretion may be prolonged.

One such infant (Figure 19) had a low birth weight (2045 g at term), microcephaly, hepatosplenomegaly, lymphadenopathy, thrombocytopenia, peripheral pulmonic stenosis, cataracts and 'blueberry muffin' skin lesions (dermal erythropoiesis) on the face, chest, abdomen and legs.

Another child had congenital rubella with similar involvement, but with a patent ductus arteriosus, and blueberry muffin skin lesions on the buttocks and leg (Figure 20). Figure 21 is an X-ray of the lower extremities of this infant and shows 'celery stalking' of the metaphyseal areas of the long bones characteristic of congenital rubella. These linear radiolucencies disappear after 2–3 months.

Cataracts (Figure 22) and glaucoma (Figure 23) presenting at birth as cloudy corneas are suggestive of congenital rubella, although other congenital infections may also cause these eye abnormalities.

Scalp abscess

Fetal monitoring with internal scalp electrodes, scalp blood sampling and trauma may result in a break in the skin with subsequent abscess formation. Group B streptococci (Figure 24), *Salmonella* species, *Escherichia coli* and *Staphylococcus aureus* are the pathogens most frequently recovered from abscesses and / or blood. Herpes simplex virus or *Neisseria gonorrhoeae* may cause infection when the mother is infected by these organisms.

This 12-day-old full-term infant with trisomy 21 (Down syndrome; Figure 25) had a cephalohematoma measuring 3 x 4 cm at birth. Delivery by low forceps was uncomplicated. Fever, lethargy, anorexia and a rapidly enlarging scalp abscess were noted on day 11 of life. A complete blood count revealed 20 000 white blood cells (WBC) / mm³ with a marked shift to the left; hemoglobin decreased from 19 g / dl to 14 g / dl, and the platelet count was 10 000 / mm³. Moderate hepatosplenomegaly persisted for 4 weeks.

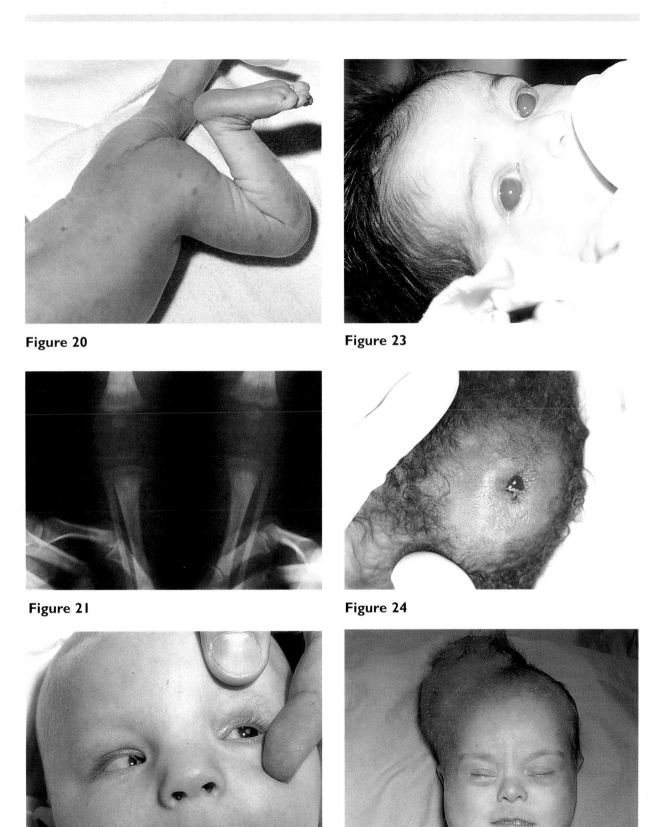

Figure 20

Figure 23

Figure 21

Figure 24

Figure 22

Figure 25

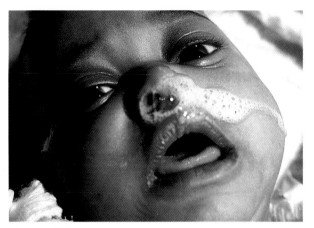

Figure 26

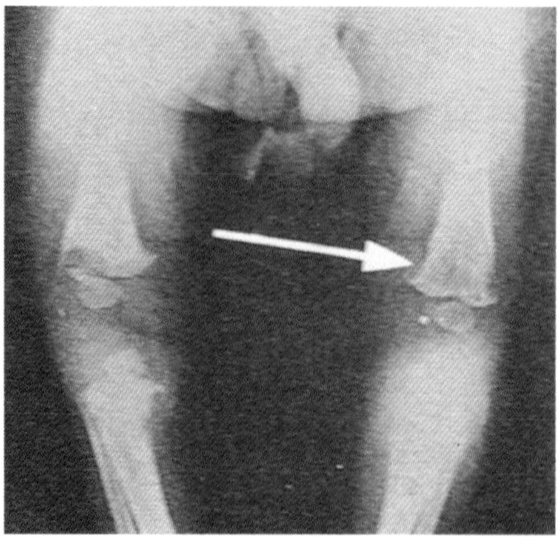

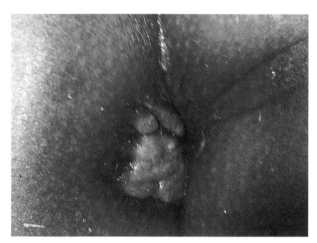

Figure 28

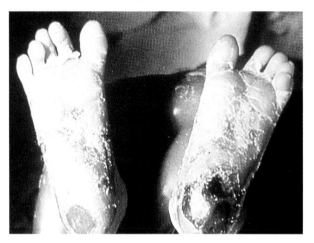

Figure 27

Figure 29

Incision and drainage produced 200 ml of purulent material with a hydrogen sulfide odor. Cultures of blood and abscess material produced a heavy growth of *E. coli*. Recovery was rapid and examination at age 2 months was normal.

Syphilis

Congenital syphilis has shown a resurgence in recent years which has been indirectly associated with the illicit-drug epidemic. Transplacental passage of this spirochete may result in fetal wastage, non-immune hydrops or postnatal manifestations such as snuffles (Figure 26), rash (Figure 27), hepatitis and osteochondritis / periostitis (Figure 28).

If syphilitic infection is left untreated, late manifestations will include neurosyphilis, deafness, and dental and bone abnormalities.

Infants infected with syphilis at birth may be asymptomatic. Evaluation of maternal serology and therapy is therefore essential to identify such infants and prevent subsequent complications. All suspect infants should be assessed for congenital syphilis initially with a non-treponemal serological test [for example, Venereal Disease Research Laboratory (VDRL) test, automated reagin test (ART) or rapid plasma reagin (RPR) test] with positive responses confirmed using a specific treponemal test [such as the microhemagglutination assay (MHA-TP) or fluorescent treponemal antibody absorption (FTA-ABS) test].

Non-treponemal tests provide quantitative titers that correlate with disease activity whereas treponemal tests provide confirmation of positive non-treponemal results and remain reactive for life despite adequate therapy. Evaluation of infants at

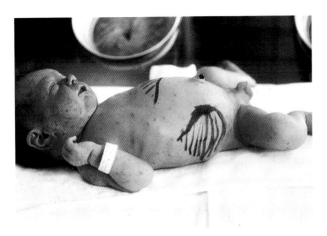

Figure 30

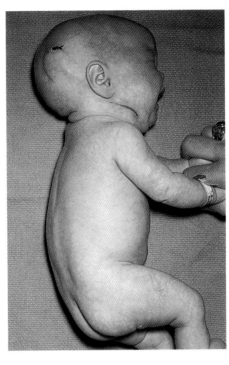

Figure 31

risk should include physical examination, non-treponemal screening assay, MHA-TP or FTA-ABS, lumbar puncture, long bone and chest X-rays. CSF findings suggestive of neurosyphilis include leukocytosis, elevated protein or a positive VDRL test.

Condyloma lata are flat moist lesions on the mucous membranes, and mucocutaneous areas of the male and female genitalia and perianal area (Figure 29). These lesions are indicative of secondary syphilis.

Dark-field examination of the condylomata and nasal secretions (see Figure 26) in this 2-month-old with congenital syphilis and snuffles showed them to be teeming with highly infectious spirochetes.

TORCH infections

Congenital infections with bacterial and non-bacterial pathogens may result in significant morbidity and mortality. TORCH, an acronym for *Toxoplasma* species, rubella virus, CMV and HSV, has become less useful with the changing incidence of common pathogens involved in congenital infections.

CMV, the most commonly implicated agent in congenital infection, is estimated to infect 1–2% of all newborns in the USA. The increased prevalence of STDs such as syphilis and HIV has resulted in increasing numbers of newborns infected with these pathogens. At the same time, screening and immunization have all but eliminated rubella as a cause of congenital infection.

Clinical manifestations of congenital infection are variable and there is considerable overlap among potential pathogens. The classical triad is jaundice, hepatosplenomegaly and a petechial rash (Figure 30). Neonates who are small for gestational age (SGA) also warrant examination for congenital infection, particularly when associated with microcephal (as in the infant with congenital rubella in Figure 19).

Toxoplasmosis

Toxoplasma gondii infection in the newborn occurs in approximately 1/1000 deliveries in the USA as a result of transplacental transmission during maternal primary infection. Most infected infants are asymptomatic at birth, but may develop symptoms later in infancy. Chorioretinitis occurs in >80% of infected infants. Other early clinical manifestations include hepatosplenomegaly, lymphadenopathy, a maculopapular or petechial rash and jaundice.

This 2-month-old (Figure 31) developed hydrocephalus, successfully controlled by a ventriculoperitoneal shunt at age 4 weeks. Skull X-rays were normal, but Gram-staining of the CSF sediment revealed *Toxoplasma* organisms. Concentrations of IgM antibody specific for *T. gondii* were elevated.

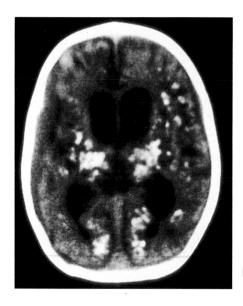

Figure 32

Computed tomography of the head at 4 months of age (Figure 32) showed marked dilatation of the ventricles with multiple calcifications and scattered hypodense areas of cerebritis. Slow motor development persisted with the infant's demise at age 14 months in spite of treatment with sulfadiazine and pyrimethamine.

Varicella–zoster

Infection *in utero* iduring primary maternal varicella (chickenpox) during the first 20 weeks of pregnancy has occasionally been reported to result in an embryopathy characterized by cicatrices and limb paralysis with atrophy. Central nervous system and eye manifestations are also described. The most critical period is 9–16 weeks of gestation. Data are not available to define the magnitude of risk, but it appears to be less than 10%.

Chickenpox in a mother beginning 5 days before to 2 days after delivery may result in severe infection in the neonate at or shortly after birth (Figure 33). Such newborns should receive varicella–zoster immune globulin as soon as possible after delivery.

When a mother has chickenpox during pregnancy, apparently unaffected neonates exposed to the virus later in life may present with unusual manifestations of the disease, as in this infant (Figure 34) who presented with vesicular lesions confined to the right lower extremity.

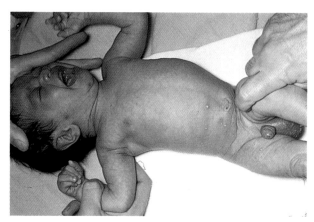

Figure 33

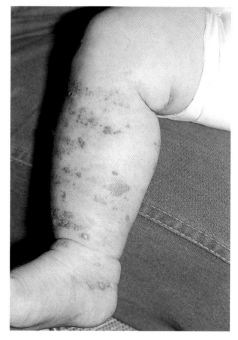

Figure 34

Infectious disease emergencies

Infant botulism

Disease in infants caused by *Clostridium botulinum* was first reported in 1976 and is now the most common form of botulism reported in the USA. The peak age of incidence is 6–8 weeks and nearly all reported cases have occurred in infants aged from 4 to 28 weeks.

Disease begins with constipation followed by poor feeding, and is frequently complicated by aspiration pneumonia and flaccid paralysis of the facial muscles. This is best appreciated when the infant is held

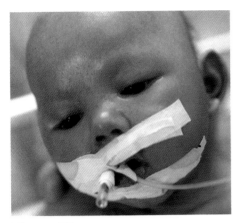

Figure 35

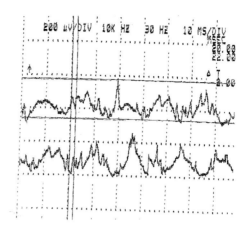

Figure 37

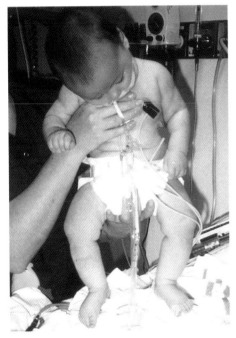

Figure 36

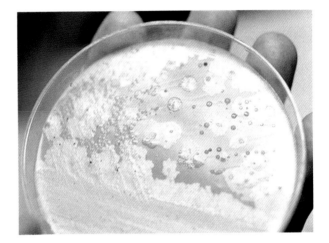

Figure 38

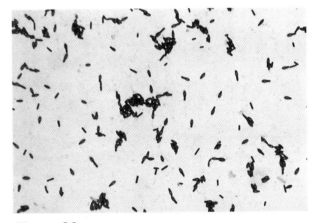

Figure 39

erect as this accentuates ptosis and causes the facial features to sag with gravity, as seen in this 6-week-old infant (Figure 35). There may also be oculomotor paralysis, with a fixed stare and widely dilated pupils followed by flaccid paralysis of the trunk and limbs (Figure 36).

Electromyography characteristically shows brief small abundant motor unit potentials (BSAP), which are considered pathognomonic (Figure 37). The definitive diagnosis is made by demonstration of *C. botulinum* toxin in the stool. *Clostridium botulinum* organisms may be recovered from the stool using a

special egg-yolk medium wherein colonies exhibit a characteristic opalescent sheen (Figure 38). Staining of these colonies reveals large Gram-positive bacilli with bulging subterminal spores, producing a 'drumstick' appearance (Figure 39).

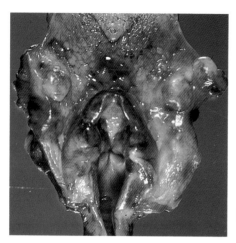

Figure 40

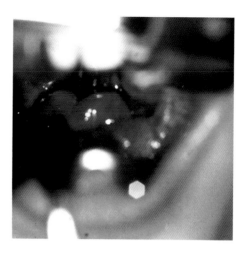

Figure 42

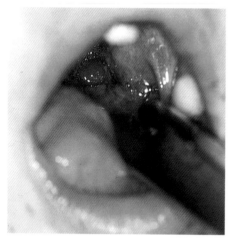

Figure 41

Severe cases require endotracheal intubation and mechanically assisted ventilation as well as parenteral hyperalimentation for up to several weeks. In the absence of cerebral hypoxemia, recovery is usually complete.

Acute epiglottitis

Fulminant infection of the epiglottis and arytenoid folds was previously caused almost exclusively by *Haemophilus influenzae* type b (Hib). The clinical course is frequently complicated by abrupt airway obstruction requiring immediate tracheostomy or endotracheal intubation for survival. Hypoxic brain damage or death will occur in a significant number of patients if infection is not recognized.

Figure 40 is an autopsy specimen from a 23-month-old boy who died in the mid-1960s, when hospitalization, intravenous antibiotics and observation were the standard of care (note the edematous and

injected epiglottis and arytenoid folds). In anticipation of such a complication, 'prophylactic' tracheotomy was proposed in the early 1970s.

Figure 41 is of an erythematous edematous epiglottis in a child with epiglotittis who required tracheostomy for abrupt airway obstruction. By the mid-1970s, prophylactic endotracheal intubation to secure the airway had become the standard of care for patients with acute Hib epiglottitis.

Figure 42 (shown here by courtesy of Dr Peter R. Holbrook) is a view of the supraglottic structures of a child with acute Hib epiglottitis in whom the airway was prophylactically secured by oropharyngeal followed by nasopharyngeal intubation. This disease has now virtually disappeared with the use of Hib protein-conjugate vaccines, first introduced in the late 1980s.

Bacterial meningitis

The clinical presentation of bacterial meningitis may only include fever, irritability or other findings indicating toxicity. The most suggestive physical feature is nuchal rigidity or a positive Brudzinski sign, elicited by rapid flexing of the neck with the child supine, hips and knees extended. With inflammation of the meninges, the patient will involuntarily flex the thigh and knees (Figure 43).

A less sensitive physical finding is the Kernig sign, which is positive when extension of the flexed knee elicits increased pain and crying. The infant in Figure 43 also has preseptal cellulitis, which is highly sug-

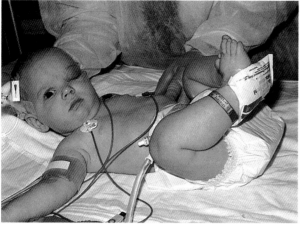

Figure 43

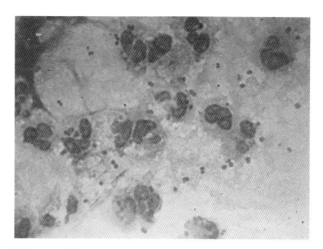

Figure 46

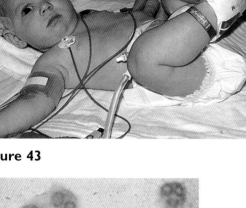

Figure 44

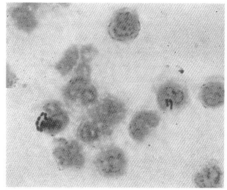

Figure 47

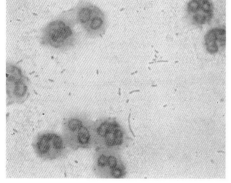

Figure 45

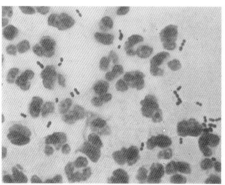

Figure 48

gestive of *Haemophilus influenzae* as the etiology. In almost all cases of preseptal or orbital cellulitis associated with meningitis, meningeal signs are present during the initial presentation. On rare occasions, however, they may not be apparent until 24 h after beginning treatment.

A Gram stain of CSF should always be performed for early identification of etiology, as this may influence the selection of initial antimicrobial therapy and decisions for adding dexamethasone during

early treatment. The reported incidences of the three most common pathogens in infants and children are currently similar and include *H. influenzae* (Figure 44), *Streptococcus pneumoniae* (Figure 45) and *Neisseria meningitidis* (Figure 46). Group B streptococci (Figure 47) remain the most common cause of meningitis in neonates, followed by *Escherichia coli* and *Listeria monocytogenes* (Figure 48). In fatal cases, gross purulence of the brain is seen at post-mortem examination, as in this neonate with *E. coli* meningitis (Figure 49).

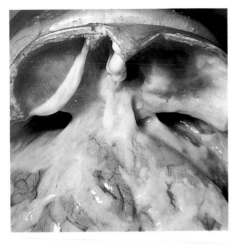

Figure 49

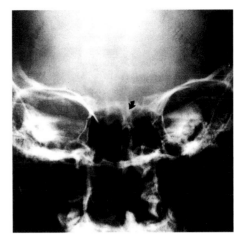

Figure 52

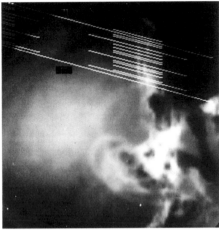

Figure 50

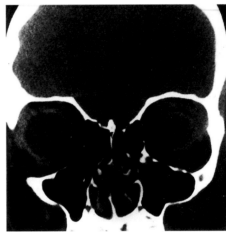

Figure 53

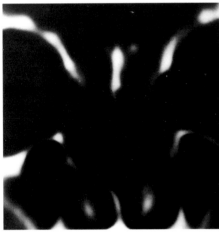

Figure 51

Recurrent bacterial meningitis

Recurrent episodes of meningitis necessitate a careful search for cranial and midline defects as predisposing factors. Plain radiography and tomography may detect only large defects, and dye or radioisotope-tracer studies using nasal packs only occasionally detect CSF leaks. Cranial CT using coronal thin-section views of the anterior cranial fossa (Figure 50) allows detailed examination of the most likely region to have an anatomical defect.

Figure 51 is a direct coronal scan of the cribriform plate region showing an osseous defect in the cribriform plate, with protrusion of a soft tissue mass (cerebral peduncle) into the nasal ethmoid region.

Coronal CT of the anterior cranial fossa (Figure 52) indicates an osseous defect (arrowed) in the cribriform plate, whereas Figure 53 is a CT of the anterior cranial fossa showing a unilateral defect in the cribriform plate with soft tissue protrusion into the ethmoid area.

Meningococcemia

Neisseria meningitidis causes illness in humans with a variety of clinical presentations, ranging from benign

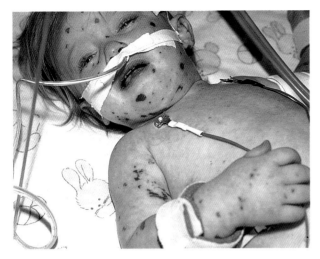

Figure 54

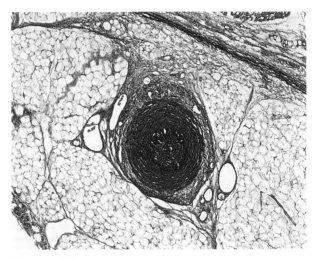

Figure 56

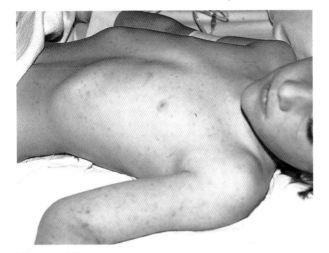

Figure 55

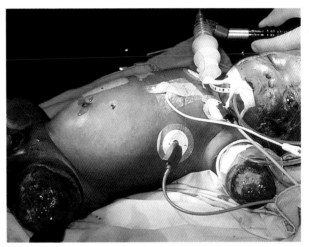

Figure 57

upper respiratory infection to acute endotoxemia. Vasculitis and chronic disease are also described. The common signs and symptoms of acute and chronic meningococcemia may initially be subtle, but fever accompanied by an ecchymotic, petechial or purpuric rash (Figure 54) should always suggest this diagnosis.

Ecchymoses are defined as non-blanching skin lesions measuring 2–10 mm. The rash may be more petechial (lesions 1–2 mm) particularly with chronic disease (Figure 55). Purpura measuring > 10 mm is associated with a poor prognosis. Disseminated intravascular coagulation and large-vessel thrombosis (Figure 56) may necessitate extensive amputation (Figure 57).

Diagnosis of meningococcemia is made by a characteristic clinical presentation and is usually confirmed by culture. Care must be taken to differentiate meningococcemia from other febrile illnesses with rashes. These include septicemia due to other bacteria (particularly *Haemophilus influenzae*), endocarditis, Rocky Mountain spotted fever and enteroviral infections.

Treatment of meningococcemia includes antibiotics and intensive supportive care when shock is present. In addition, prophylactic treatment of family members and other close contacts of the index case is indicated, using rifampin, ciprofloxacin or, for pregnant women, ceftriaxone.

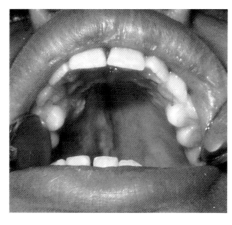

Figure 58

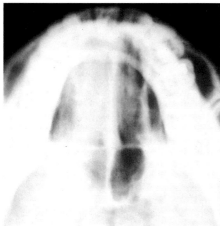

Figure 59

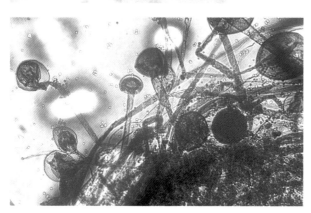

Figure 60

Mucormycosis

Acute rhinocerebral mucormycosis is diagnosed most frequently in patients with insulin-dependent diabetes or immunodeficiency and has a high mortality. Illness begins with pain, swelling and tenderness at the site of primary infection. Necrotic lesions appear in the nasal cavity or palate (Figure 58). Hemorrhage into these lesions results in a characteristic black discoloration (not seen in this patient). Infection may rapidly destroy bone in the sinuses (Figure 59) and extend into the central nervous system. Thrombosis of the cavernous sinus or internal carotid artery may also occur.

Diagnosis is made by tissue biopsy showing nonseptate, irregularly branching, hyphal forms of *Rhizopus oryzae* (Figure 60), *R. rhizopodoformis* or other members of the order Mucorales.

Necrotizing fasciitis

Classification of necrotizing soft-tissue infections is based on the anatomical structures involved, the pathogens recovered and the clinical presentation. Bacteriologically speaking, there are two distinct types of necrotizing fasciitis: type I is polymicrobial and involves synergistic interactions among bacteria to produce an aggressive destructive infection; type II is caused by group A beta-hemolytic streptococci alone or in combination with *Staphylococcus aureus*.

In neonates, *Escherichia coli* is a common single pathogen, as in this 6-day-old infant whose skin discoloration progressed in just over 5 h from an area measuring 2 x 1 cm to involve the entire chest and abdomen (Figure 61). Treatment is radical surgical debridement of all devitalized tissue (Figure 62) and appropriate antibiotics.

Purpura fulminans

Disseminated intravascular coagulation (DIC) may produce thrombocytopenic purpura with hemorrhagic infarction and necrosis of the skin. This often fatal process is seen most frequently in children and is precipated by severe infection caused by streptococci, meningococci, varicella–zoster, measles or rickettsiae. In addition, protein C and protein S deficiencies can cause similar disease in neonates.

The primary pathology is a consumptive coagulopathy of plasma coagulation factors (fibrinogen factors II, V and VIII) with associated thrombocytopenia, hypofibrinogenemia and hypoprothrombinemia. Even with early treatment of the infection and correction of clotting-factor deficiencies, the mortality rate is 20%.

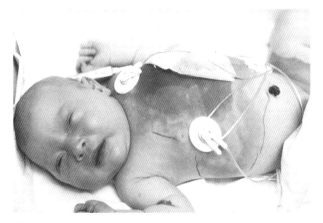

Figure 61

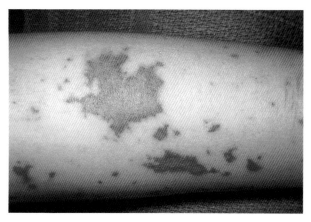

Figure 64

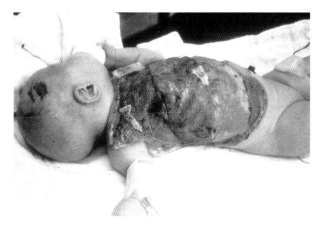

Figure 62

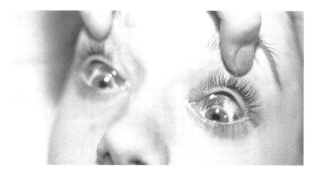

Figure 65

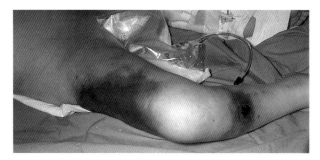

Figure 63

This 3-year-old girl with hemorrhagic chickenpox developed purpura fulminans associated with group A beta-hemolytic streptococcal bacteremia (Figure 63). Her leukocyte count was 50 000/mm³ with a hemoglobin of 6 g/dl. Platelet count was also 50 000/mm³. Recovery was complete following penicillin therapy.

This 4-year-old developed DIC with extensive purpura on the third day of sepsis and meningitis

caused by *Neisseria meningitidis* (Figure 64). Recovery after penicillin therapy was complete without sequelae.

Staphylococcal toxic shock syndrome (Staph-TSS)

Epidemic Staph-TSS occurred in the USA in association with the introduction and use of hyperabsorbable and occlusive vaginal tampons in the late 1980s. These products were withdrawn from the market and the incidence of menstrual-associated disease decreased dramatically. However, sporadic cases of menstrual- and non-menstrual-associated Staph-TSS continue to be reported.

The site of infection is usually superficial. There is a characteristic prodrome of high fever, headache, sore throat, abdominal pain and severe vomiting with watery diarrhea. This is followed by increasing toxicity and, after 24–48 h, marked non-suppurative conjunctival injection often with hemorrhage (Figure 65), with hyperemia of the oral mucosa and

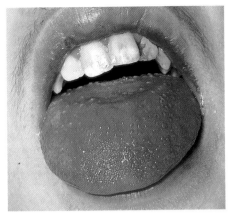

Figure 66

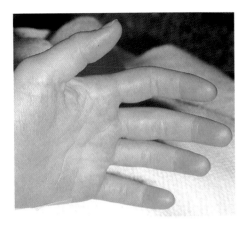

Figure 70

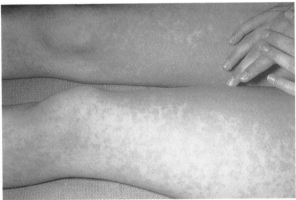

Figure 67

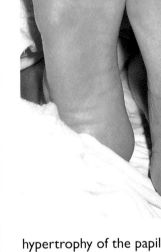

Figure 71

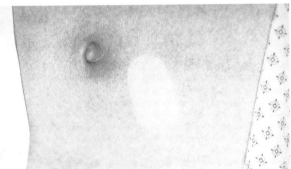

Figure 68

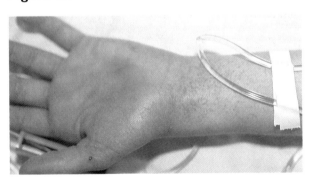

Figure 69

hypertrophy of the papilla of the tongue (Figure 66) similar to that seen in scarlet fever and Kawasaki syndrome. This is soon followed by a sunburn-like erythematous macular rash, which usually starts on the trunk and becomes generalized.

Figures 67 and 68 show erythroderma and delayed capillary filling. Petechiae occur especially around the wrists and ankles (Figure 69), and shiny edema of the hands (Figure 70) and feet (Figure 71) may be seen. Postural hypotension ensues, associated with confusion and lethargy, and followed by shock, multiple organ failure and death in 5–10% of patients if early treatment is not provided. Erythroderma fades after 2–4 days, and full-thickness desquamation of the hands (Figure 72) and feet (Figure 73) occurs after 1–2 weeks.

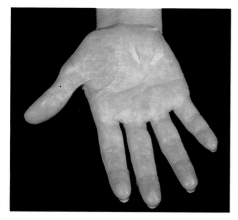

Figure 72

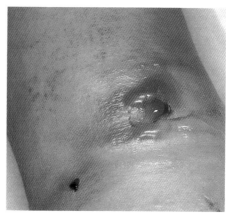

Figure 75

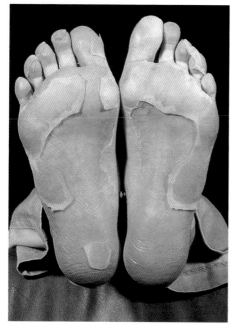

Figure 73

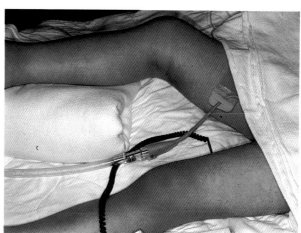

Figure 76

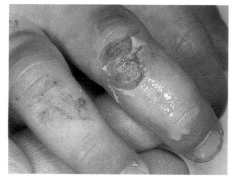

Figure 74

Streptococcal toxic shock syndrome (Strep-TSS)

This is caused by toxin-producing strains of invasive group A beta-hemolytic streptococci (GABHS). The disease is characterized by a vague prodrome

of increasing deep painful swelling and tenderness in an extremity over 2–3 days following injury to the area. Abrupt onset of fever, rigors, toxicity and shock may occur with rapid development of multi-organ failure. Mortality has varied from 30 to 50% primarily due to delay in diagnosis and treatment.

This 4-year-old girl initally had an abscess on her finger (Figure 74; shown here by courtesy of Dr Martin E. Weisse). Four days later (3 days prior to hospitalization), she fell and hurt her right shoulder, producing pain and swelling which persisted for 2 days. Several hours prior to hospital admission, she developed a vesiculobullous lesion in the right ante-cubital area (Figure 75), high fever, rigors, toxicity, lethargy, shock and cardiopulmonary arrest.

The child was treated with antibiotics, fluid resusci-tation, intubation and assisted ventilation. A gener-alized erythematous rash developed over 24h (Figure 76) and subsided over the next 2–3 days

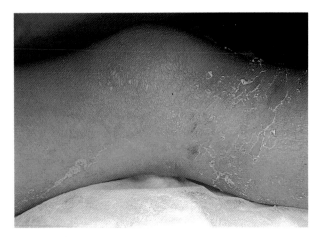

Figure 77

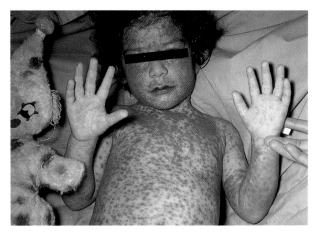

Figure 80

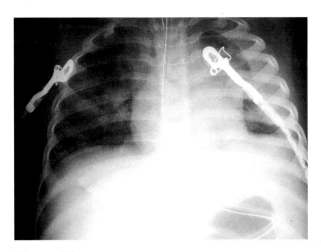

Figure 78

Figure 79

complete blood count (CBC), urinalysis and chest radiograph. The patient became pallid, then ashen, followed by cardiorespiratory arrest while being sponged with water to reduce the fever. Intubation, ventilation, fluid resuscitation, ionotropic therapy and parenteral antibiotics were provided, but the child remained anuric with poor cardiac output.

Left lower lobe pneumonia with effusion developed over several hours (Figure 78) and a Gram stain of the pleural fluid showed Gram-positive cocci in chains (Figure 79). GABHS grew on culture. The child developed multiple organ failure including shock-lung and died 18 h after hospital admission (30 h after onset of illness).

Maculopapular exanthematous diseases

Drug eruptions

Antibiotics, analgesics, anticonvulsants, and various food substitutes and flavorings are often implicated as causing allergic skin rashes in children. Fixed drug eruptions characteristically recur in the same site and are discrete oval or round infiltrative lesions, varying from 0.5 to several centimeters in size. Purpura with vesicles and / or bullae may be seen. Pruritus is minimal or absent. Lesions persist for 1–3 weeks with spontaneous resolution after removal of the offending agent.

followed by desquamation 7–10 days later (Figure 77). GABHS was cultured from the blood obtained on admission.

A 22-month-old boy with fever of up to 40.5 °C lasting 12 h showed a normal initial examination,

This fixed drug eruption in a 3-year-old (Figure 80) was due to clindamycin and / or ampicillin, which

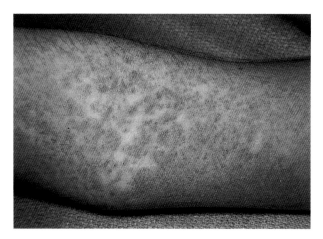

Figure 81

had been taken on several occasions. A similar rash had been observed 1 year previously.

Phenytoin is associated with a particularly high incidence of drug eruptions. This 11-year-old (Figure 81) presented with a pruritic maculopapular scarlatiniform generalized eruption of 11 days' duration. Persistent fever, sore throat, generalized lymphadenopathy and aphthous mouth ulcers were found. CBC showed leukocytosis with 43% atypical lymphocytes.

Enteroviral infections

Enteroviruses, a subgroup of picornaviruses, are a common cause of exanthems in children. These viruses (poliovirus, coxsackievirus, echovirus and reovirus) spread by contact from person to person, and initiate infection in the oropharynx before attacking the gastrointestinal tract. The rash is usually generalized, non-pruritic and maculopapular, but may be vesicular, scarlatiniform, zosteriform, urticarial, petechial or purpuric. The majority of these eruptions persist for 2–8 days.

A typical example of the pruritic maculopapular eruption is shown in this 11-year-old, who had no other symptoms (Figure 82). No medications had been taken. Examination was normal except for the generalized rash which was also on the palms and soles. The rash cleared spontaneously in 8 days.

This enanthem (Figure 83), characterized by aphthous ulcers on the soft palate (herpangina), in a 15-

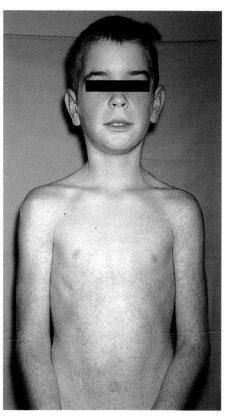

Figure 82

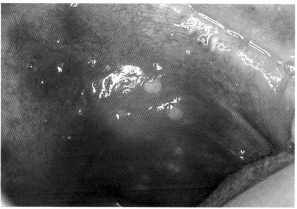

Figure 83

year-old with a generalized maculopapular rash, fever, sore throat and tender anterior cervical lymph nodes is most compatible with coxsackie A virus infection.

Epstein–Barr virus (EBV)

The infectious mononucleosis syndrome characterized by fever, sore throat, fatigue, malaise and generalized lymphadenopathy is associated with EBV, although adenovirus, CMV, *Toxoplasma gondii*, viral

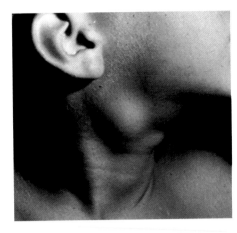

Figure 84

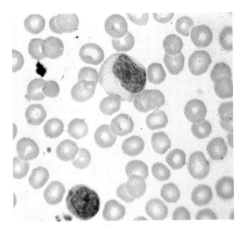

Figure 86

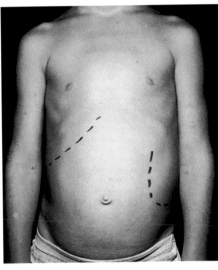

Figure 85

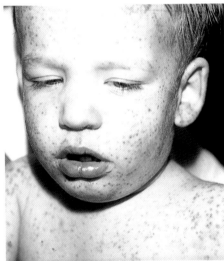

Figure 87

hepatitis, HIV and drug hypersensitivity may occasionally produce a similar illness.

This previously healthy 9-year-old developed fever, a generalized papular rash, sore throat, dysphagia, arthralgia and abdominal pain. Lymphadenopathy (Figure 84), hepatosplenomegaly (Figure 85) and exudative tonsillitis were noted. CBC showed 34 000 leukocytes / mm^3 with 37% atypical lymphocytes and abundant cytoplasm (Downey cells; Figure 86). A monospot test was positive and a four-fold rise in EBV-specific serology confirmed the diagnosis. Spontaneous recovery occurred within 3 weeks.

In a younger patient, amoxicillin for 3 days was ineffective and, in fact, accentuated the rash into a widespread pustular dermatitis (Figure 87). Note the eyelid edema and petechiae on the ear lobes, both of which are characteristic of infectious mononucleosis.

EBV infection may also cause a spectrum of oncological processes, such as Burkitt's lymphoma, nasopharyngeal carcinoma, Hodgkin's disease and lymphoproliferative disorders, especially in patients with immunodeficient states and / or AIDS.

Erythema infectiosum

Parvovirus B19 infection in children usually presents as a mild exanthematous illness termed erythema infectiosum (also called fifth disease). It begins with a distinctive 'slapped cheek' red rash lasting 1–3 days, followed by a generalized maculopapular exanthem of 7–10 days' duration. The rash may increase in intensity, producing a lace-like appearance, during periods of increased physical activity, exposure to sunlight or high environmental temperature. Fever occurs in 15–30% of patients during the first 2 days of illness, and arthralgia is common in adult women.

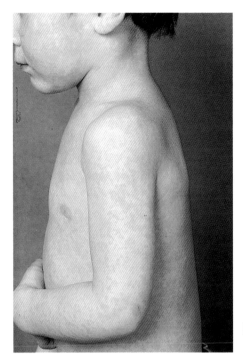

Figure 88

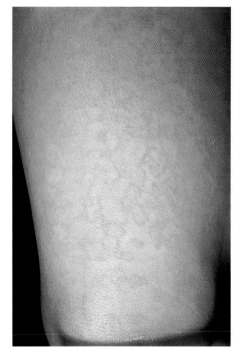

Figure 89

Parvovirus B19 infection may also produce a mild respiratory illness, arthritis in adults, chronic anemia in immunodeficient patients and an aplastic crisis in patients with chronic hemolytic anemias.

This 4-year-old presented with a fever and non-pruritic rash for 2 days (Figure 88). The cheeks were intensely red and a diffuse maculopapular rash persisted for 10 days. During the next 3–4 weeks, a transient lace-like rash (Figure 89) was noted for several hours during increased physical activity.

Erythema multiforme minor

Erythema multiforme (EM) is a distinct hypersensitivity syndrome of unknown pathogenesis, characterized by unique skin and mucous membrane lesions. Infectious agents are the most common precipitating etiologies. EM can be differentiated from urticaria by the primary skin lesions. In EM, all lesions appear within 72 h and remain in a fixed location for at least 7 days. Papules, usually totalling over 100, evolve into target lesions with central vesicles, bullae or crusts. Itching or burning of individual lesions occurs, but is rarely severe.

EM due to coxsackie A virus was diagnosed in this 15-year-old with a 6-day history of a generalized

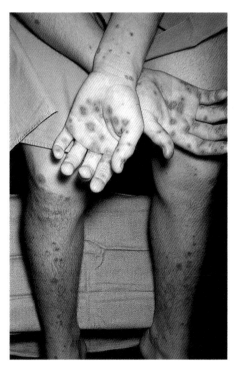

Figure 90

pruritic erythematous rash, and tender mouth and hands. Tetracycline had been taken for 4 days and 'allergy pills' for 2 days. Examination was normal except for multiple fixed iris and circular macules, with central target red-purple lesions particularly concentrated on the extremities (Figure 90). Vesicopustules were seen in the mouth, and on the

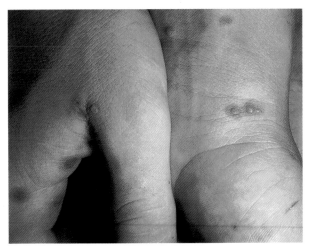

Figure 91

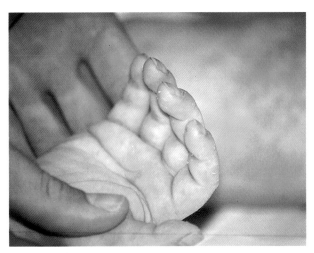

Figure 93

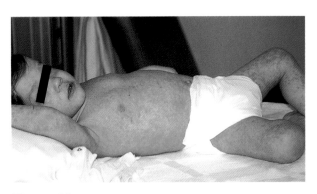

Figure 92

fingers (Figure 91), ankles and feet. Spontaneous resolution occurred within 2 weeks.

Kawasaki disease

Because there is no definitive laboratory test for identifying Kawasaki disease, diagnosis depends on the presence of five of six clinical features (Figure 92), including:

(1) Bulbar conjunctivitis

(2) An enanthem of erythematous mouth and pharynx, strawberry tongue and red cracked lips

(3) A generalized erythematous rash

(4) Extremity changes, such as swelling or erythema

(5) Adenopathy, with one cervical node > 1.5 cm in diameter

(6) Fever lasting more than 5 days.

Other features include sterile pyuria, arthritis, arthralgia, carditis and gallbladder hydrops. Following the acute phase, desquamation of the fingertips (Figure 93) or hands and feet is characteristic. Coronary aneurysms represent the most serious consequence of this disease (Figure 94) as death may result from occlusion subsequent to thrombus formation or progressive artery stenosis. High-dose intravenous immunoglobulin in conjunction with aspirin decreases the incidence of coronary artery disease.

Measles

Rubeola or measles begins with a prodrome of increasing fever, clear rhinorrhea, photophobia and cough of 2–5 days' duration. A rash then develops on the face along the forehead and in front of the ears, and soon involves the whole of the face with conjunctival injection (Figure 95). Rhinorrhea and cough worsen, and there may be epiphora.

Koplik's spots appear on the buccal mucosa opposite the upper and lower premolar teeth (Figure 96) 24–48 h before onset of the rash, and may persist for 48–72 h after onset of the rash. If the spots are not present 24 h before and after onset of the rash, then the diagnosis of measles in unlikely.

On the first day of the rash, reddish-purple macules 3–7 mm in diameter coalesce on the face and shoulders to become confluent (Figure 97). On the second day, the rash appears on the shoulders (Figure

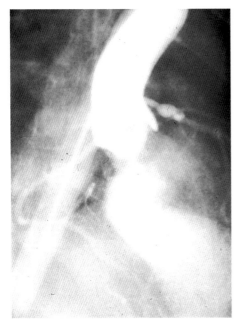

Figure 94

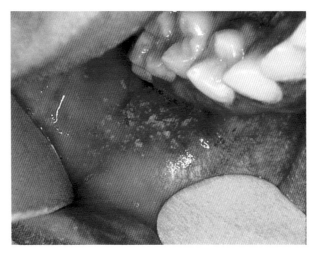

Figure 96

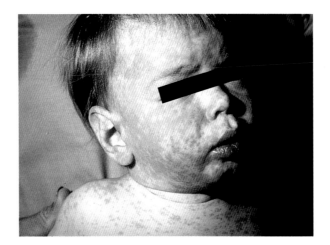

Figure 97

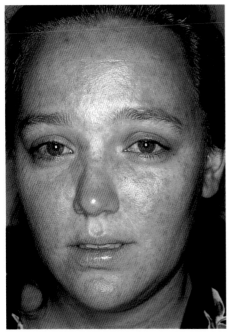

Figure 95

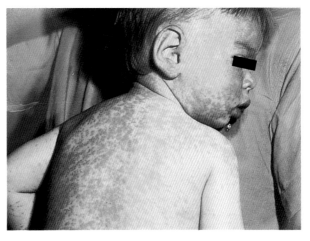

Figure 98

98) and trunk and, by the third day, spreads to the thighs. At this time, the rash on the face fades, leaving a fine white powdery desquamation. Fever and rhinorrhea subside, but the cough persists for 1–2 weeks.

Patients who received killed measles-virus vaccine when it was available during 1963–68 are only partially protected from infection. (By definition, these patients would now be adults.) Once exposed to the natural virus, the disease assumes an atypical presentation (atypical measles), with a centrifugal

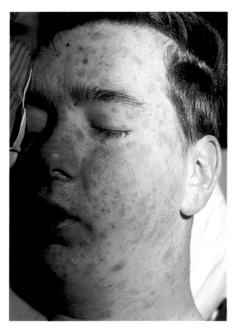

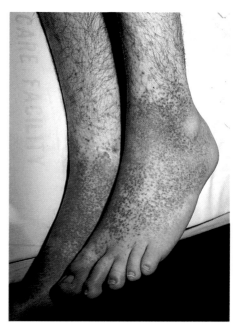

Figure 99

Figure 100

maculopapular to petechial rash (Figures 99 and 100) following a prodrome of high fever, headache, abdominal pain and myalgia. A non-productive cough associated with pleuritic chest pain is commonly seen as a consequence of pneumonia and often with a pleural effusion. Evolution of the rash is variable. Only the distal extremities are involved in some patients whereas, in others, the trunk as well as entire extremities are affected. Patients with atypical measles are not considered contagious.

Roseola infantum

Human herpesvirus 6 (HHV-6) was first isolated in 1986 from cultures of patients with lymphoreticular disease. This herpesvirus group is ubiquitous. By 3 years of age, most children have been infected. HHV-6 has two subgroups: A and B. No disease is presently associated with group A whereas group B appears to be the major etiological agent of roseola, also called sixth disease or exanthem subitum.

Infection is characterized by 3–5 days of high fever with a paucity of physical findings. The temperature rapidly returns to normal, at which time a morbilliform rash appears. Figure 101 demonstrates roseola in a 7-month-old infant whose rash was preceded by 3 days of temperatures up to 104 °F and irritability, but otherwise normal findings on physical examination. On the fourth day, the patient

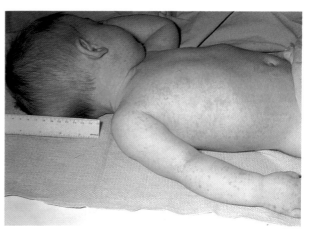

Figure 101

was afebrile with an extensive generalized maculopapular rash and bilateral 10-mm suboccipital nodes. The rash faded within 48 h.

Rubella

Rubella, a togavirus, usually causes a mild 3-day illness. Clinical features are minimal with low-grade fever, a fine discrete maculopapular rash and generalized lymphadenopathy, particularly cervical, postauricular and / or suboccipital. Transient polyarthralgia and polyarthritis occasionally occur in children, but are common in female adolescents and adults. Encephalitis and thrombocytopenia are rare complications.

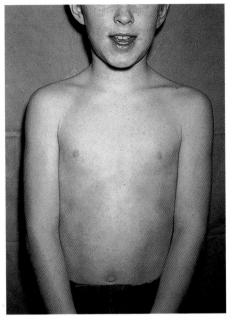

Figure 102

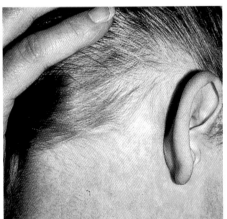

Figure 103

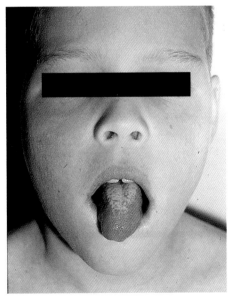

Figure 104

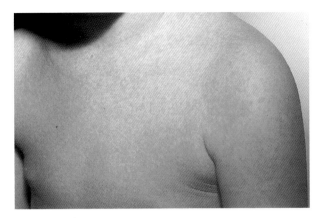

Figure 105

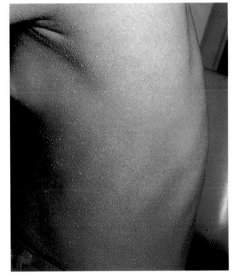

Figure 106

This 9-year-old child (Figure 102) developed low-grade fever and a non-pruritic generalized, discrete, maculopapular eruption, which resolved spontaneously within 72 h. Another child of the same age also had postauricular adenopathy (Figure 103).

Scarlet fever

Scarlet fever occurs with pharyngitis or wound infections due to erythrotoxigenic GABHS in individuals who have not had prior exposure to the toxin. The rash starts on the neck, axillae and shoulders, and is usually faint on the face, where a malar flush with circumoral pallor may be more evident (Figure 104).

The rash is most pronounced on the trunk, appearing as a generalized sunburn-like erythroderma (Figures 105 and 106). There is a palpable sand-

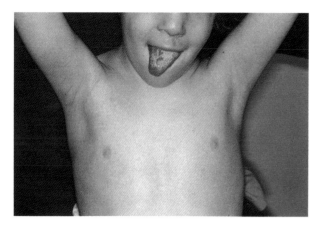

Figure 107

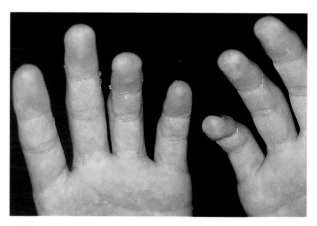

Figure 109

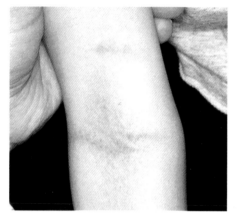

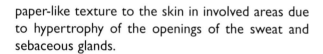

Figure 108

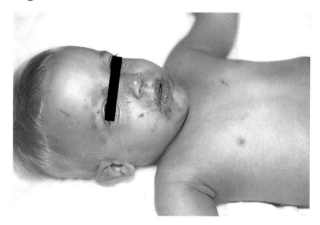

Figure 110

paper-like texture to the skin in involved areas due to hypertrophy of the openings of the sweat and sebaceous glands.

The hallmark of the rash of scarlet fever is the marked intensity of the rash in the flexural creases; this is most apparent in the axillae and groin (Figure 107), but is also seen in the antecubital areas where the darkened creases are called Pastia's lines (Figure 108). The erythroderma begins to fade after 2–3 days and a generalized desquamation, starting with the hands (Figure 109) and feet, occurs after 7–10 days. (Figures 104–109 are shown here by courtesy of Dr Martin E. Weisse).

Staphylococcal scalded skin syndrome (SSSS)

This term refers to a spectrum of dermatological disorders caused by a soluble exotoxin produced by certain strains of *Staphylococcus aureus*. The most severe form is Ritter's disease, in which there is a

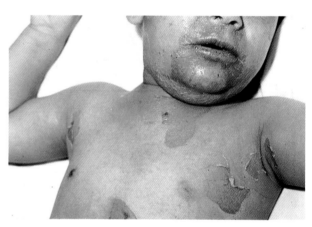

Figure 111

bullous desquamation of large areas of skin in neonates. This is called toxic epidermal necrolysis (TEN), or Lyell's disease in older children or adults, although the etiology is more likely to be idiopathic or secondary to drug hypersensitivity. More common is a diffuse scarlatiniform erythroderma (Figure

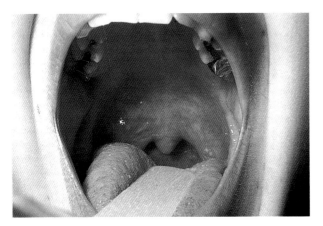

Figure 112

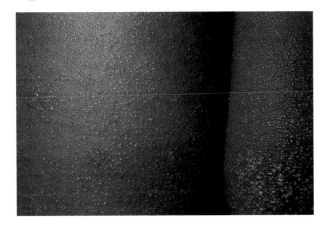

Figure 113

110), which progresses to desquamation of involved areas and a positive Nikolsky sign (Figure 111).

In the USA, most of the exotoxin-producing staphylococci belong to phage group II. The characteristic histopathological feature is a cleavage plane high in the epidermis with no inflammatory reaction.

Papulovesicular exanthematous diseases

Coxsackievirus infections

Human enteroviruses include 23 which are classified as coxsackie A viruses and six which are coxsackie B. In infants and young children, these viruses are responsible for frequent and occasionally significant disease although, most usually, the illness is non-specific and febrile. Other less common, but more serious, diseases are seen in the summer and

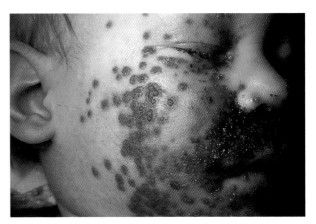

Figure 114

fall, and involve one of the following organ systems:

(1) Upper and lower respiratory tract: common cold, pharyngitis, herpangina, stomatitis, pneumonia and pleurodynia

(2) Gastrointestinal: vomiting, diarrhea, abdominal pain and hepatitis

(3) Eye: acute hemorrhagic conjunctivitis

(4) Heart: myopericarditis

(5) Skin: exanthems

(6) Neurological: aseptic meningitis, encephalitis and paralysis.

Figure 112 shows coxsackievirus A 9 infection in an 18-year-old with fever, severe sore throat, multiple oropharyngeal vesicopustular lesions, and a maculopapular rash of the head, neck and trunk. Spontaneous recovery occurred within 6 days.

Figure 113 shows coxsackievirus A 5 illness in a 6-year-old with malaise, headache, coryza, fever, generalized adenopathy, hepatosplenomegaly and a maculopapular rash. The rash became papulovesicular on day 5, but resolved spontaneously with fine desquamation and complete recovery by day 7.

Eczema herpeticum

Cutaneous dissemination of herpes simplex virus (HSV) type 1 or 2 in patients with atopic eczema or chronic dermatitis is termed eczema herpeticum or Kaposi's varicelliform eruption. Figure 114 shows an example of extensive HSV infection on the face of a 14-month-old infant with atopic dermatitis. The

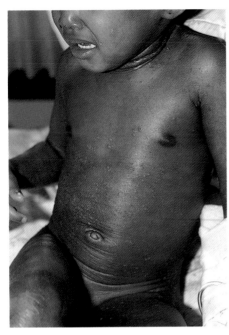

Figure 115

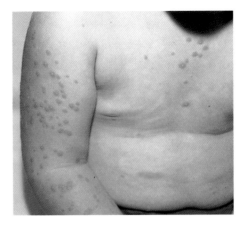

Figure 117

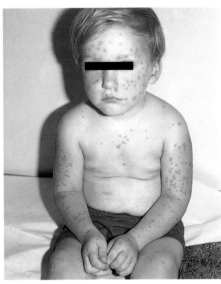

Figure 116

HSV dermatitis cleared spontaneously within 14 days without treatment.

The disease is variable, ranging from mild self-limiting lesions to rapidly fatal infection. Extensive vesicular and crusting eruptions may result in painful weeping with excessive fluid loss and bacterial superinfection (Figure 115). Patients usually have high fever and are irritable.

Severe manifestations are associated with deficient cell-mediated immunity, such as in the Wiskott–Aldrich syndrome. In limited trials, both intravenous

and oral acyclovir have been shown to control progression of the disease. The differential diagnosis includes eczema with secondary bacterial infection and varicella.

Gianotti–Crosti syndrome

Also known as papular acrodermatitis of childhood, this disease is characterized by the rapid development of symmetrical flat-topped (lichenoid) skin-colored or erythematous papules in a centrifugal distribution (Figures 116 and 117). It is self-limiting, but lasts for 3–6 weeks.

One-quarter of these cases are associated with hepatitis B, as in this child (Figure 116) who had hepatomegaly, elevation of liver enzymes and positive serology for hepatitis B surface antigen. Most cases in children are anicteric. Outbreaks have been reported with EBV infection and case reports suggest that this rash is also a manifestation of AIDS.

Other viral agents which produce this rash include parainfluenza and coxsackie A16 viruses. The peak age of incidence is 1–6 years with a 2:1 male to female predominance. These cutaneous changes are presumed to be a reaction to either viral or immune-complex deposition.

Herpetic whitlow

Primary cutaneous herpes may be found anywhere, but is particularly common in children who suck their thumbs or fingers, with inoculation and as a secondary infection of the digits. The lesion is a painful vesicular eruption. Where the diagnosis is

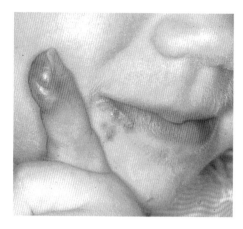

Figure 118

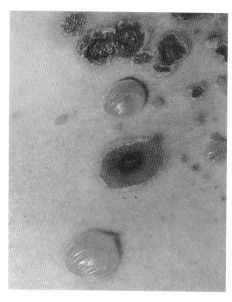

Figure 121

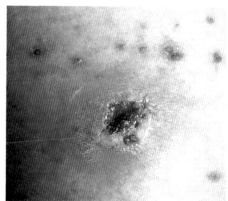

Figure 119

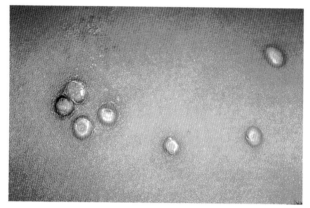

Figure 122

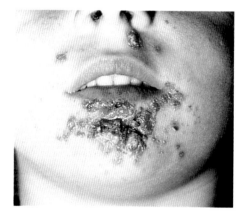

Figure 120

not clinically apparent, Tzanck test preparations, fluorescent staining for herpes or viral cultures may be performed on scrapings of the lesions. Figure 118 shows herpetic whitlow in a child with recurrent herpes simplex labialis.

Impetigo

This term refers to superficial infection of the skin which may be primary or secondary to abrasions and insect bites. Impetigo lesions are classified as pustular (Figure 119), honey-crusted (Figure 120) or bullous (Figure 121). The latter is due almost exclusively to *Staphylococcus aureus*. Prior to 1980, impetigo was caused primarily by GABHS and, although *S. aureus* was also frequently implicated, treatment with penicillin alone was sufficient. Subsequently, however, penicillin-resistant *S. aureus* has evolved as the major cause of impetigo. Treatment with an oral macrolide, a penicillinase-resistant penicillin, a cephalosporin or a topical antibiotic provide optimal treatment.

Molluscum contagiosum

Poxvirus infection of the skin is manifested by single or multiple raised, firm, smooth, waxy, skin-colored, flat or umbilicated tumors which vary in size from 1 to several millimeters in diameter (Figure 122).

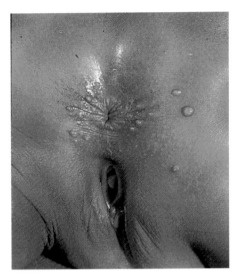

Figure 123

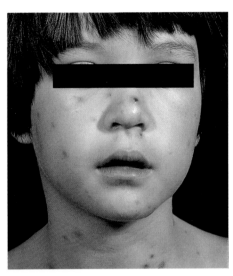

Figure 126

These lesions occur primarily in children and tend to resolve spontaneously over several months. Numerous molluscum lesions in the anogenital area (Figure 123) may be the result of child abuse.

Papular urticaria

This common childhood eruption is a sensitivity reaction to insects such as fleas, mosquitoes and chiggers. Children usually present in the spring or summer with multiple bites and/or papules and wheals on all extremities and, to a lesser extent, on the face, trunk and buttocks.

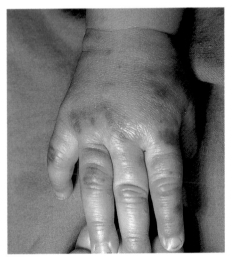

Figure 124

The rash comprises numerous urticated papules 3–10 mm in diameter with occasional wheals, some with a central hemorrhagic punctum. Because pruritus is usually present, scratching produces secondary excoriation, inflammatory ulcerations and impetiginized crusts. If insect bites are subsequently avoided, most lesions resolve within 10–21 days, but may persist for months or even years if the child is re-exposed to insect bites.

This 7-month-old presented with pruritic papules and wheals on all extremities for several days (Figure 124). The mother noted a daily variation in the intensity of the rash from one extremity to another. When purpuric face lesions appeared and itching persisted, consultation was requested.

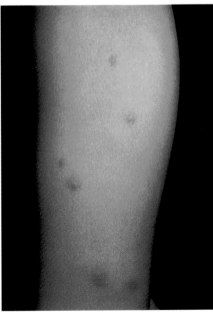

Figure 125

Examination revealed multiple purpuric and inflamed papules and wheals on all extremities, and

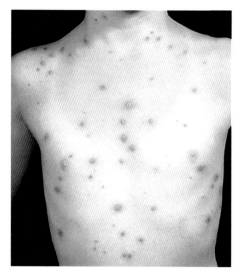

Figure 127

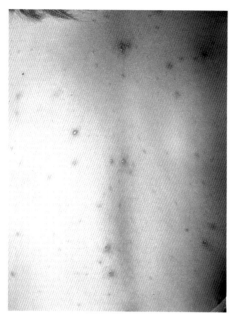

Figure 128

similar lesions on the face. The family dog was treated for fleas and the infant treated with diphenhydramine. The rash resolved within 17 days.

This 5-year-old presented with a similar history of multiple inflamed papules and wheals on all extremities (Figure 125). Pruritus was moderate. All lesions resolved within 2 weeks with diphenhydramine therapy and elimination of cat fleas.

Varicella–zoster

Primary varicella is referred to as chickenpox whereas exacerbation of latent infection is termed herpes zoster or shingles. Varicella lesions first appear on the face (Figure 126) and along the hairline, then spread to the trunk within 1–2 days (Figure 127).

Although varicella skin lesions vary in form from erythematous macules to papules, vesicles and pustules, the classic diagnostic lesion is the uniloculated vesicle on an erythematous base (Figure 128), also described as a 'dew-drop on a rose petal'. Crops of macules, papules, vesicles and pustules are all frequently seen in the same area at the same time (Figure 129), and continue to evolve and resolve over several days, after which only desquamating scales and scabs are seen.

Fever and systemic symptoms vary with the severity of the rash, but most patients have only a few skin lesions, and are afebrile and asymptomatic.

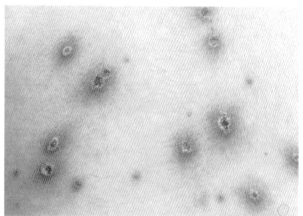

Figure 129

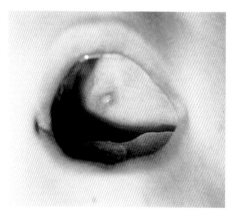

Figure 130

Approximately one-quarter have an enanthem which is manifested as ulcerative lesions on the oral mucosa (Figure 130).

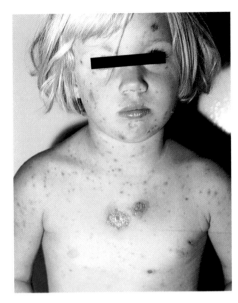

Figure 131

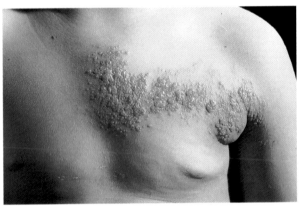

Figure 132

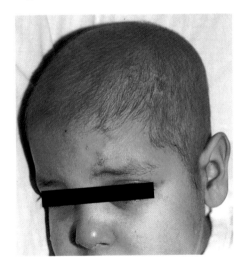

Figure 133

The most common complication of varicella is secondary infection of the lesions, most often due to GABHS (Figure 131). Although apparently trivial,

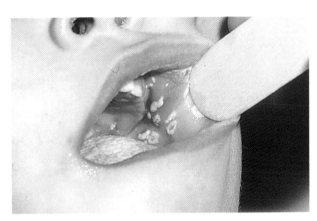

Figure 134

these infections may progress to severe invasive disease (see streptococcal toxic shock syndrome).

Herpes zoster usually occurs in subjects with a history of mild varicella at a young age or where previous infection was subclinical. It begins with hyperesthesia or pain along a neurocutaneous pathway on the trunk (Figure 132) or on a branch of the trigeminal nerve (Figure 133). The lesions typically appear in clusters of vesicles on an erythematous base arranged in a linear dermatone distribution.

Enanthems

Candidiasis

Thrush is the common term used to describe oral candidiasis, manifested by the presence of irregular white plaques on the tongue, buccal mucosa, lips and palate (Figure 134). Gram-staining shows large Gram-positive budding yeast forms with pseudohyphae (Figure 135).

The peak incidence of thrush occurs in infants during the first 2–3 months of life but may be seen in otherwise healthy children at up to 1 year of age. Candidiasis may also be seen in older children who have been treated with broad-spectrum antibiotics. Severe and persistent oral candidiasis suggests an underlying immunodeficiency.

Cyclic neutropenia

Defective maturation of uncommitted stem white blood cells results in an absolute neutropenia which

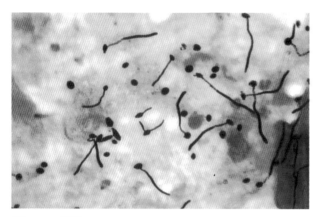

Figure 135

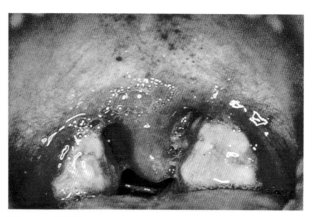

Figure 137

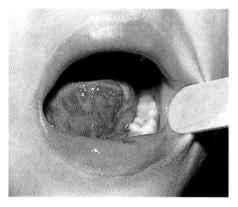

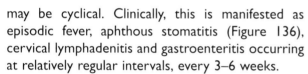

Figure 136

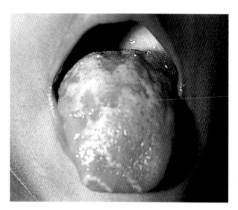

Figure 138

may be cyclical. Clinically, this is manifested as episodic fever, aphthous stomatitis (Figure 136), cervical lymphadenitis and gastroenteritis occurring at relatively regular intervals, every 3–6 weeks.

Signs and symptoms are usually not evident until the neutrophil count has already begun to rise. Diagnosis therefore requires quantitation of white blood cell concentrations in blood during the period immediately preceding anticipated clinical events. Some patients may also have similar cyclical fluctuations in erythrocytes and platelets.

Treatment includes aggressive oral hygiene, antibiotics during febrile or symptomic episodes and granulocyte-colony stimulating factor (G-CSF) for more severe infectious complications.

Exudative tonsillopharyngitis

Almost all upper respiratory tract infections are caused by viral agents and require only symptomatic therapy, as in this teenager (Figure 137) whose

pharyngitis was caused by EBV. Note the petechiae on the soft palate. As pharyngitis or tonsillitis without nasal involvement is more commonly associated with group A streptococci, a throat culture or test for streptococcal antigen is essential for determining this bacterial etiology. Often, documentation of an outbreak of oropharyngeal infection caused by a particular viral pathogen will provide guidance to the management of subsequent cases.

Rare, but important, bacterial pathogens that cause pharyngitis are *Arcanobacterium hemolyticum*, *N. gonorrhoeae*, *Corynebacterium diphtheriae* and *Francisella tularensis*, with other groups of streptococci, particularly C and G, accounting for isolated outbreaks of disease.

Geographical tongue

Also known as benign migratory glossitis and occasionally confused with an infectious enanthem, this (Figure 138) is found in 1–2% of the population, especially in those who are atopic.

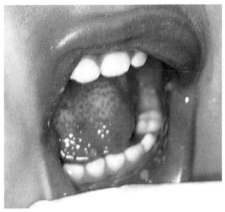

Figure 139

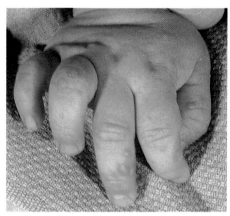

Figure 140

Contrasting regions on the dorsum of the tongue account for the unique appearance of irregular red patches, with loss of filiform papillae, surrounded by elevated grayish-white exudative borders that change in configuration from day to day.

This congenital developmental anomaly requires no treatment. Similar benign anomalies include fissured or scrotal tongue and median rhomboid glossitis.

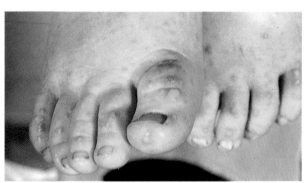

Hand–foot–mouth disease

Figure 141

Coxsackieviruses A16, A5, A9, A10, B1 and B3 may produce a low-grade fever, headache and vesicular lesions in the mouth, hands and feet which last for 3–10 days, occasionally with associated aseptic meningitis. The mouth lesions are yellowish ulcers with erythematous borders on the tongue, lips, gums, buccal mucosa and palate (Figure 139). Skin lesions comprise erythematous macules, papules and vesicles on the hands (Figure 140) and feet (Figure 141) and, less commonly, on the buttocks. Lesions on the hands and feet are oval with the long-axis lying parallel to the dermal ridges. Some lesions may appear pustular (Figure 142).

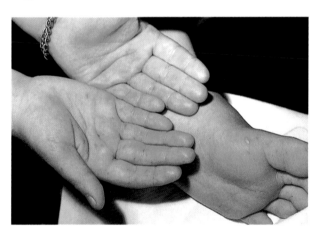

Figure 142

Hand–foot–mouth disease should be differentiated from primary herpetic gingivostomatitis in which gingivitis, fever and cervical lymphadenopathy are prominent.

Herpangina

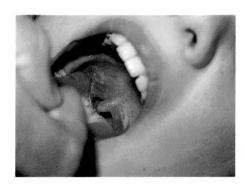

One or more oral yellowish ulcers several millimeters in diameter, with surrounding erythematous rings measuring an additional 4–6 mm in diameter, is

Figure 143

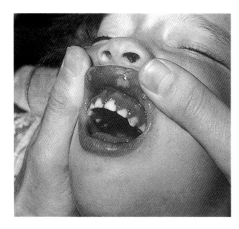

Figure 144

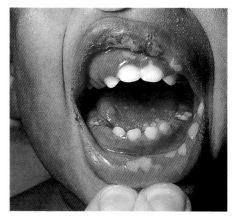

Figure 145

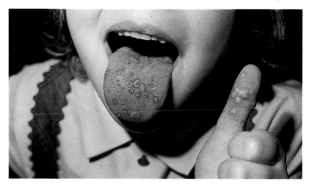

Figure 146

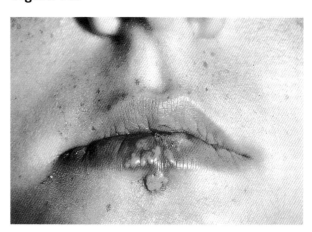

Figure 147

characteristic of herpangina. Lesions are most often seen on the anterior tonsillar pillar (Figure 143), less often on the uvula and soft palate, and rarely on the posterior pharyngeal wall. Lesions are not seen anterior to these areas. There may be mild-to-moderate fever, sore throat, irritability and feeding difficulty in young infants, and headache and malaise in older children.

Herpangina is caused by infection by a number of coxsackieviruses (both A and B) and echoviruses. The disease usually lasts only 3–6 days. Some cases may have associated aseptic meningitis.

Herpes gingivostomatitis

Primary herpetic gingivostomatitis (PHGS) occurs in children aged between 6 months and 3 years who present with yellowish ulcers that are one to several millimeters in diameter on the gums, gingiva, buccal mucosa, lips, tongue and palate, most with surrounding rings of erythema (Figure 144). The lesions are not seen in the posterior mouth or pharynx, but there may be a preceding exudative tonsillopharyngitis without mouth lesions, particularly in older children and adults.

The gingiva are frequently edematous with a purplish erythema, and are tender, painful and friable with a tendency to bleed when touched (Figure 145). In older children who are thumb-suckers, PHGS may be associated with secondary herpetic whitlow (Figure 146).

Most children with PHGS have mild-to-moderate fever and anterior cervical lymphadenopathy. The disease usually lasts only 4–7 days, but may persist for 1–2 weeks. Some foods and juices may cause pain when taken, but most children are able to take milk and milk products, including ice cream, to maintain adequate hydration and nutrition.

As the primary infection subsides, the virus establishes a latent infection in the trigeminal ganglia for life and may express exacerbation as recurrent herpes labialis infections or 'fever blisters' (Figure 147).

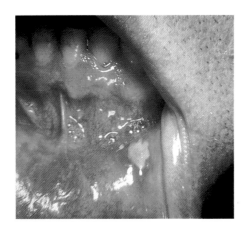

Figure 148

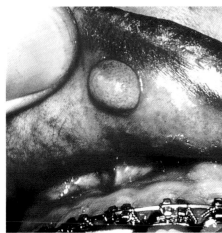

Figure 149

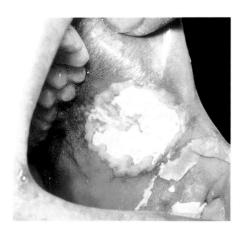

Figure 150

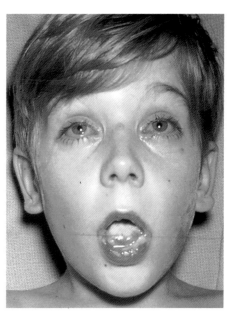

Figure 151

The cause of aphthae is likely to be minor oral trauma with subsequent bacterial overgrowth, as lesions are more common in children fitted with braces or other orthodontic devices. With chronic trauma, the lesions may form fibrosing mucoceles (Figure 149) adjacent to the ducts of minor salivary glands.

Treatment is rarely necessary except when lesions are extensive or severe. Light cauterization with silver nitrate is advocated by many dermatologists, but aggressive cauterization can result in significant damage to the mucosa (Figure 150).

Stevens–Johnson syndrome (SJS)

Erythema multiforme major or SJS is a severe bullous form of erythema which presents with acute onset of high fever and pronounced systemic symptoms. Two or more mucous membranes, usually the mouth and eyes, are initially involved with lesions, followed by the genitalia, perineal and nares.

SJS lasts 2–6 weeks, depending on the causative agent, which is usually infectious (HSV, EBV, measles virus, *Mycoplasma*) or drugs (anticonvulsants, sulfonamides, non-steroidal anti-inflammatory drugs). HSV infection accounts for 80% of childhood cases. Ocular changes (keratitis, uveitis, severe conjunctivitis, corneal ulceration, panophthalmitis) may result in partial or complete blindness. Photophobia

Recurrent aphthae

Single or multiple shallow ulcers which periodically develop on the gums, tongue, palate, oropharynx and buccal mucosa opposite the biting surface of the teeth (Figure 148) are variously called recurrent aphthae, aphthous stomatitis, or aphthae. The term aphthous stomatitis has also been used synonymously with herpetic gingivostomatitis.

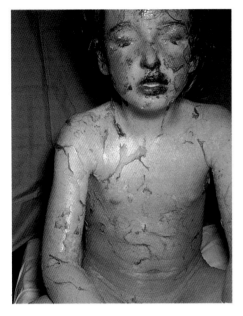

Figure 152

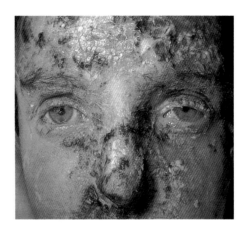

Figure 153

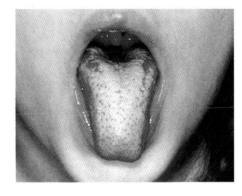

Figure 154

may be severe and persistent. A mortality of 5% is reported in children in contrast to 15% in adolescents and adults.

SJS due to *Mycoplasma pneumoniae* occurred in this 11-year-old (Figure 151) who developed cough and coryza for several days, followed by acute-onset fever, malaise, severe cough and headache. Multiple target lesions appeared rapidly over the trunk and extremities, with severe conjunctivitis and exudative dermatitis of the lips, tongue and, subsequently, the entire oral cavity.

Chest X-ray revealed bilateral pneumonitis. Oral erythromycin therapy effected a prompt decrease in fever, cough and malaise, leading to complete recovery after 11 days.

This 8-year-old developed an extensive generalized erythematous dermatitis with high fever, malaise, anorexia, photophobia, exudative stomatitis and conjunctivitis 10 days after measles was diagnosed (Figure 152). The rash progressed rapidly over 12 h to multiple vesicobullae, with pruritus and extensive peeling of the skin.

In spite of high-dose prednisone therapy (60 mg/day), there was generalized desquamation with continuation of fever and malaise. Oral and ocular lesions persisted with severe stomatitis, conjunctivitis and photophobia.

By day 18, the skin was healing, but corneal clouding, thinning and corneal ulcerations developed (Figure 153). Over the next 6 weeks, the disease slowly resolved. After 2 months, the skin and oral mucosa were normal. However, the patient had persistent keratitis and photophobia with total blindness due to corneal opacification.

Strawberry tongue

This appearance (Figure 154) is associated with scarlet fever (see Figures 104–109). The tongue and oral mucosa are hyperemic, and there is hypertrophy of the papillae of the tongue. There may be a partial white coat which, after 2–3 days, desquamates to leave a raw uncoated 'raspberry tongue'.

Vincent's gingivostomatitis

Gingival infection with necrosis involving the interdental papillae and gums is referred to as acute necrotizing gingivitis, trench mouth or Vincent's gingivostomatitis (Figure 155). When tonsillar tissue is also involved, use of the term 'Vincent's angina' is more appropriate.

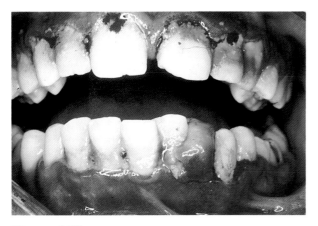

Figure 155

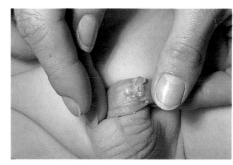

Figure 157

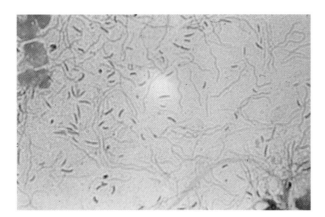

Figure 156

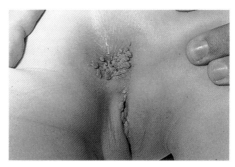

Figure 158

The causal organisms are *Borrelia* species (Figure 156) and other penicillin-sensitive fusiform bacilli and spirochetes. In developing countries and historically throughout much of the world, infection was related to malnutrition and poor oral hygiene. Currently, this disease is more commonly a consequence of cytolytic chemotherapy in cancer patients, with tissue breakdown in the mouth and secondary overgrowth of colonizing microflora.

Sexually transmitted diseases

Condylomata acuminata

Also known as genital warts, these irregular raised verrucous lesions are often seen on the mucous membranes and mucocutaneous areas of the genitalia (Figure 157) and perineal areas (Figure 158), but rarely on the mucous membranes of the mouth. The disease is caused by human papillomaviruses, predominantly types 6 and 11. Incubation may be

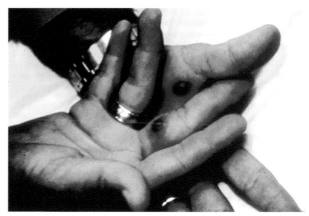

Figure 159

prolonged so that lesions in infants and children who are up to 2–3 years of age may have been acquired perinatally. Condylomata acuminata in older children suggests childhood sexual abuse.

Gonococcal infection

Most uncomplicated gonococcal infections (gonorrhea) produce symptoms of urethritis in adolescent males whereas disease in females is frequently asymptomatic. Disseminated gonococcal infection (DGI) following bacteremia often produces petechial or pustular acral skin lesions that begin to appear 3–21 days after exposure together with asymmetrical arthralgias, tenosynovitis or septic

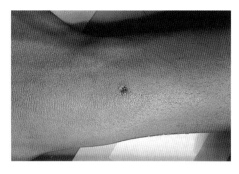

Figure 160

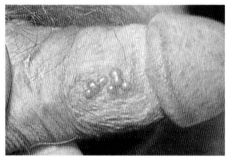

Figure 161

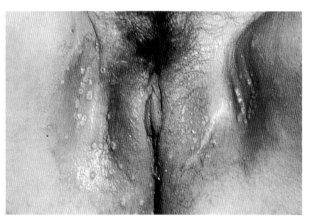

Figure 162

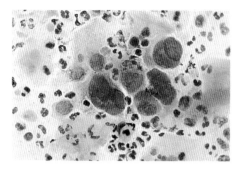

Figure 163

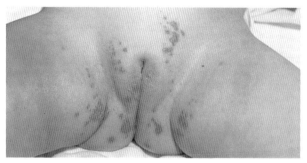

Figure 164

arthritis. This is referred to as the arthritis-dermatitis syndrome (Figure 159).

Other manifestations of DGI are hepatitis, endocarditis and meningitis. Diagnosis of uncomplicated gonorrhea in males can be made by Gram-staining of the urethral discharge with demonstration of Gram-negative intracellular diplococci (see Figure 2) whereas culture is required in females.

A sexually active 15-year-old girl (Figure 160) presented with fever, chills and arthralgia, and several papular lesions over the face and extremities. Cultures of blood, cervix and skin pustules were negative for *N. gonorrhoeae*. However, punch biopsy

of a pustule was positive for diplococci on immunofluorescent analysis. Parenteral ceftriaxone therapy effected prompt recovery.

Genital herpes simplex

Most cases of genital herpes (herpetic vulvovaginitis and herpes progenitalis) are caused by herpes simplex virus serotype 2 (HSV-2). Infection is usually asymptomatic, although HSV is recognized to be the most common etiology of genital ulcers. Lesions can be painful.

This typical herpes progenitalis penile ulcer (Figure 161) in a teenager healed spontaneously without antiviral therapy. HSV-2 vulvitis (Figure 162) and cervicitis with perineal dermatitis were diagnosed in an 18-year-old adolescent. A smear of the cervical vesicles (Tzanck preparation) revealed multinucleated giant cells with intracytoplasmic inclusions and eosinophilic intranuclear inclusions (by Papanicolaou stain; Figure 163).

Infection may also occur in young children, transmitted from the contaminated hands of caregivers or during sexual abuse. This 8-month-old infant has HSV-2 diaper dermatitis (Figure 164) which resolved spontaneously in 12 days without sequelae.

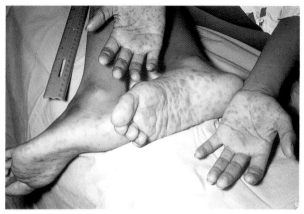

Figure 165

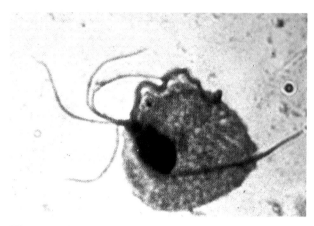

Figure 167

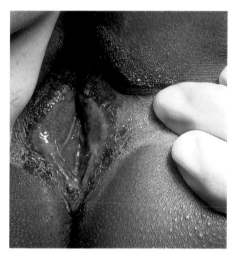

Figure 166

Syphilis

Syphilis caused by the *T. pallidum* spirochete has continued to be a hidden epidemic among adolescents and young adults. Asymptomatic disease is twice as common in 15–19-year-old females as in males in this age group.

There are three clinical stages: primary, with mucocutaneous (genital, anal, oral) painless ulcers; secondary, with a maculopapular exanthem involving the palms and soles, and generalized lymphadenopathy, fever, malaise, arthralgia, splenomegaly and genital or perianal condylomata lata; and tertiary or latent (>6 months–>2 years), with neurosyphilis and/or rarely cardiovascular or gummatous disease. Moth-eaten alopecia may be seen in the secondary stage. Diagnostic tests include screening non-treponemal (VDRL, RPR, ART) and specific treponemal (FTA-ABS, MHA-TP) tests.

Secondary syphilitic copper-colored papulosquamous rash lasting 1 week was seen on the palms and soles of this 9-year-old girl (Figure 165) following sexual abuse. Examination revealed a vaginal chancre (Figure 166) containing numerous *T. pallidum* organisms on dark-field examination. VDRL test was positive and penicillin therapy effective.

Trichomoniasis

Trichomonas vaginalis is a flagellated protozoan (Figure 167) whose presence is often asymptomatic in females. Moderate-to-heavy colonization produces a yellow-green discharge with a pH >4.5 and a fishy odor associated with pruritic vaginitis, cervicitis or urethritis. Infection in postmenarchal girls strongly suggests sexual activity whereas, in premenarchal children, trichomoniasis necessitates careful examination for sexual abuse.

Diagnosis is made by direct microscopic examination (wet preparation) of fresh vaginal discharge. Males are more frequently symptomatic with urethritis or prostatitis.

Vaginosis

Bacterial vaginosis, also called non-specific vaginitis, results from the overgrowth of *Gardnerella vaginalis* and/or anaerobes such as *Mobiluncus* species. The diagnosis is suggested by the presence of a homogeneous discharge (Figure 168) with a pH >4.5 and a positive amine odor test. More specific is the presence of clue cells (Figure 169), epithelial cells containing clumps of bacteria on their surface.

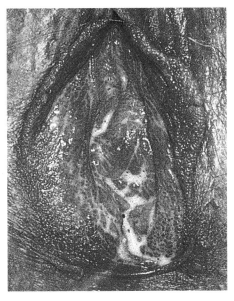

Figure 168

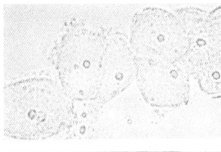

Figure 169

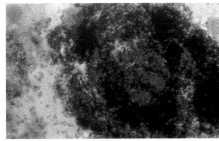

Skin, soft tissue and lymph node infections

Abscesses

Boils or furuncles (Figure 170) are the major manifestation of *S. aureus* infections when they occur in the skin. Multiloculated furuncles are called carbuncles. Group A beta-hemolytic streptococci are often associated with abscesses in the head and neck areas, and Gram-negative enteric bacilli are implicated as the cause of abscesses on the abdomen and pelvis, particularly on perianal and perirectal areas (Figure 171).

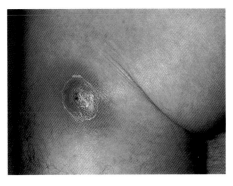

Figure 170

Actinomycosis

The four most common clinical presentations of infection with *Actinomyces israelii* are cervicofacial ('lumpy-bumpy jaw'; Figure 172), abdominal, thoracic/mediastinal and pelvic. Pathogenesis is presumed to begin with mucous membrane trauma in patients with poor oral hygiene, aspiration into the lung of endogenous flora of the oral cavity or perforation of an abdominal hollow viscus such as a ruptured appendix.

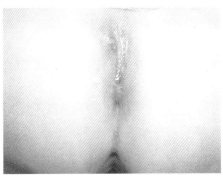

Figure 171

Pelvic disease is usually associated with the presence of an intrauterine device. The disease is chronic, with sites of infection containing polymorphonuclear leukocytes and monocytes/macro-

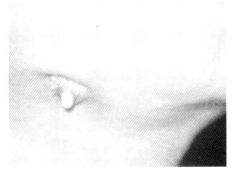

Figure 172

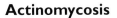

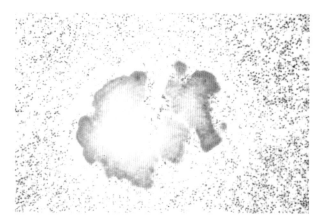

Figure 173

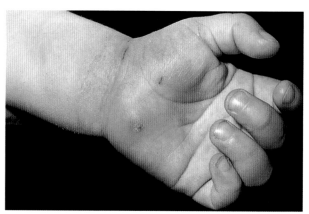

Figure 175

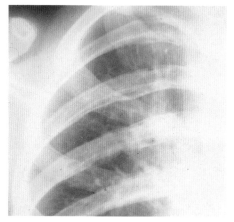

Figure 174

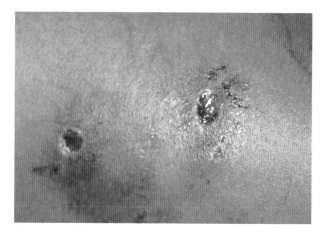

Figure 176

phages together with characteristic sulfur granules (Figure 173). Material for microscopic examination is best obtained from purulent sinus-tract drainage. Pulmonary actinomycosis may dissect into the mediastinum to produce an abscess with involvement of the adjacent ribs (Figure 174).

Animal bites

Punctures are more likely to become infected than tears or open lacerations. As most cat bites result in punctures, they have a high rate of infection (30–50%) whereas dog bites, which usually result in tears or lacerations, have low infection rates (6–10%).

Infection following both cat and dog bites is usually due to *Pasteurella multocida*, although *Staphylococcus aureus* and *S. intermedius* are also frequent pathogens. Infection with *P. multocida* is apparent as early as 12 h after a bite, with swelling, redness and

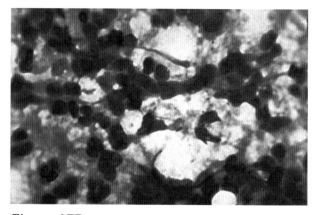

Figure 177

tenderness around the puncture marks (Figure 175, a cat bite; Figure 176, a dog bite).

Staining of purulent discharge from these lesions may reveal Gram-negative bacilli (Figure 177). Dog bites, and rarely cat bites, may become infected with *Capnocytophaga canimorsus*, which is associated

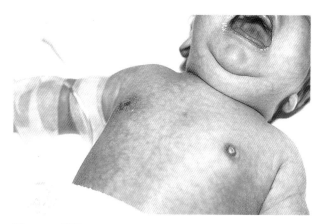

Figure 178

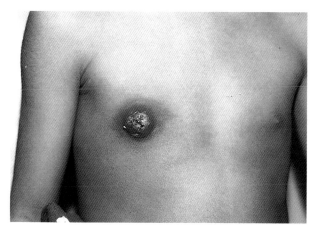

Figure 179

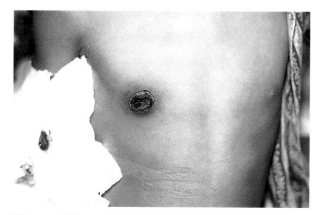

Figure 180

with a high incidence of septicemia and death in asplenic and immunocompromised patients.

Breast abscess

Coagulase-positive staphylococci account for 90% of breast abscesses. The majority are seen in

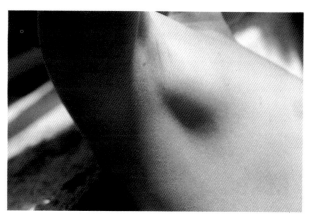

Figure 181

neonates during the first 2 weeks of life (Figure 178) in association with physiological breast enlargement, but infection may occur at any age in girls. As with other staphylococcal soft-tissue infections, the prominent feature is abscess formation with a minimal surrounding cellulitis (Figure 179). Fever and constitutional symptoms are rarely present.

Surgical drainage is required for cure as inadequate treatment may result in destruction of the breast bud and cosmetically unacceptable reduction in ultimate breast size. In this case (Figure 180), the breast bud was identified and preserved during surgery while the abscess was drained.

Cat-scratch disease (CSD)

Bartonella henselae is the cause of CSD, which usually presents with chronic adenopathy or chronic lymphadenitis (Figure 181) >3 weeks following exposure to kittens. This boy had a fever of up to 104°F, with headache, anorexia, fatigue, tender axillary lymphadenitis and a 9-lb (4.08-kg) weight loss over 7–10 days. He had allowed a kitten to sleep in bed with him and thus received multiple scratches. A crusted primary inoculation papule on his upper chest was noted 4 weeks prior to his illness. A CSD skin test produced a 30-mm area of induration. The adenitis resolved spontaneously within 4 months.

CSD is the most common cause of Parinaud's oculoglandular syndrome, a combination of conjunctivitis and preauricular adenitis. This 7-year-old suffered a corneal abrasion while playing with a pet cat. The injury produced a conjunctival granuloma

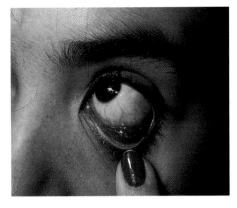

Figure 182

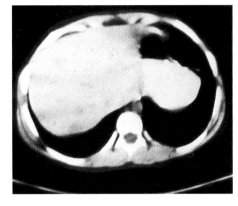

Figure 184

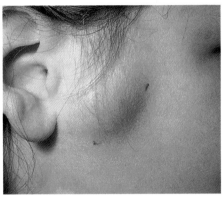

Figure 183

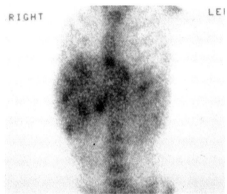

Figure 185

persisting 3–4 weeks (Figure 182). Parotid gland swelling (Figure 183) due to intraparotid adenopathy was present for 2–3 months.

CSD can also cause multifocal hepatosplenic abscesses and encephalitis. A 3-year-old had high fever for 16 days, anorexia and lethargy, with cervical adenopathy and splenomegaly. Multiple kitten scratches had produced papules on both arms that appeared 2 weeks prior to the illness. The family cat had five kittens which were heavily flea-infested.

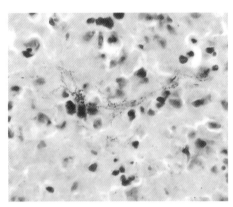

Figure 186

Ultrasonography and CT revealed multiple hypoechoic defects in the liver and spleen (Figure 184). The erythrocyte sedimentation rate was 90 mm / h. An indirect fluorescent antibody titer for *B. henselae* was 1:8193; a CSD skin test resulted in a 22-mm area of induration.

Five days after ciprofloxacin treatment began, the patient was admitted to hospital with recurrent grand mal seizures and fever. Recovery was rapid with a normal neurological examination 7 days later. Repeat ultrasound scans of the liver and spleen were normal.

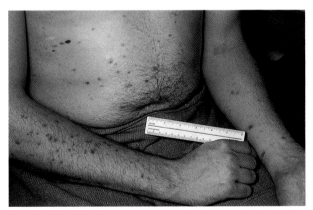

Figure 187

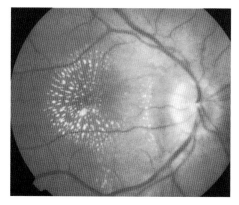

Figure 188

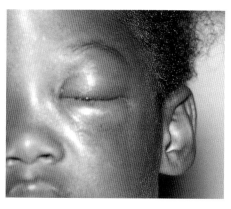

Figure 191

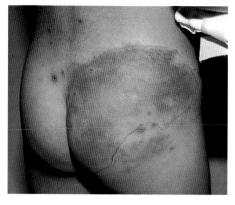

Figure 189

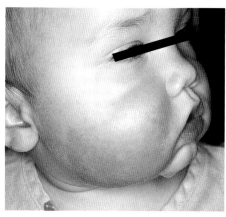

Figure 190

Examination of the right fundus revealed papilledema with a macular star and retinal white spots (Figure 188). Visual acuity was 20 / 50. The left fundus was normal. A CSD skin test resulting in a 35-mm area of induration confirmed the diagnosis. Spontaneous resolution of adenopathy and return of normal vision occurred in 3 months, and the maculopapular rash resolved in 6 months.

Cellulitis

Infection of the skin and subcutaneous tissue is manifest by spreading erythema and edema with a well-defined margin usually from a point source, frequently an abrasion, insect bites or, as in Figure 189, an infected varicella lesion. Group A beta-hemolytic streptococci are the likely pathogens especially when the cellulitis appears to originate from a point source on the skin.

Buccal cellulitis due to *Haemophilus influenzae* type b, or Hib (Figure 190), was a well-recognized form of cellulitis before the routine administration of Hib conjugate vaccines in the late 1980s. Hib cellulitis occurs primarily in infants and young children, most of whom are febrile and bacteremic. The cellulitis arises in areas with intact overlying skin presumably as a result of the bacteremia.

At present, *Streptococcus pneumoniae* is the most common etiology of periorbital (preseptal) cellulitis which occurs as an extension of sinus infection (Figure 191). CT of the orbits shows a diffuse swelling of tissues in the preseptal area with normal retro-orbital anatomy (Figure 192).

A gallium scan of a similar patient showed multiple areas of increased uptake in the liver (Figure 185). Liver biopsy revealed a granuloma containing CSD bacilli, identified with a Warthin–Starry silver stain (Figure 186).

This young man (Figure 187) had flu-like symptoms for 3 weeks prior to experiencing decreased vision in his right eye. A papular rash was noted on his abdomen and arms that was attributed to flea bites and cat scratches. Other findings were submental adenopathy and splenomegaly.

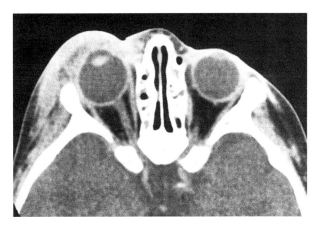

Figure 192

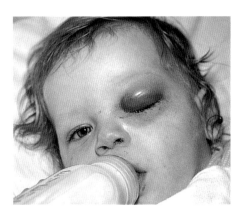

Figure 193

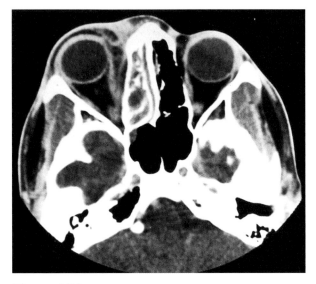

Figure 194

In contrast, this child with orbital or postseptal cellulitis (Figure 193) had Hib bacteremia. CT of the orbit (Figure 194) shows opacification of the right ethmoid sinuses with subperiosteal abscess formation in the right retro-orbital space, and displacement of the eye and orbit contents forwards to produce proptosis.

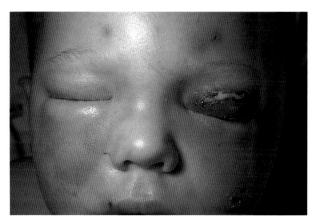

Figure 195

Erysipelas

This is superficial cellulitis of the skin with marked lymphatic vessel involvement caused by group A beta-hemolytic streptococci (GABHS). The face and scalp are most often infected following a break in the skin. A small area of redness gradually enlarges into a hot, painful, shiny bright-red, well-demarcated plaque with surrounding edema and induration.

While recovering from chickenpox, this 2-year-old boy developed acutely tender, red, swollen skin over both cheeks and the nasal bridge (Figure 195) after having scratched his left upper eyelid. Three days later, there was facial edema, fever to 106 °F and irritability. The patient experienced a generalized seizure 1 day prior to admission. Culture of the eye exudate produced a heavy growth of GABHS. Oxacillin therapy was effective with recovery in 48 h. Culture of the mother's finger pustules also grew GABHS.

This 5-month-old infant had erysipelas (Figure 196) which was associated with otitis media and GABHS bacteremia.

Erysipeloid

This teenager was injured by a catfish spike while cleaning the fish. A localized painful cellulitis was noted 2 days later (Figure 197). *Erysipelothrix rhusiopathiae* was cultured from a soft-tissue biopsy.

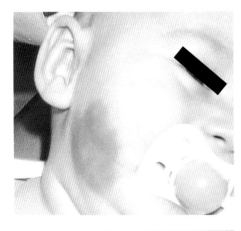

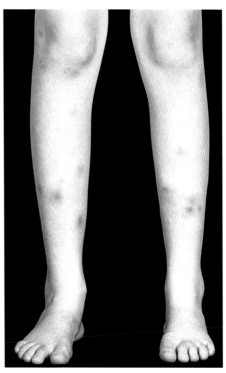

Figure 196

Figure 199

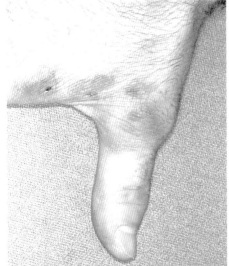

This organism is a commensal colonizing bacteria of many animal species, which renders contact with wild game or handling foodstuffs the usual risk factor for humans.

Figure 197

Absence of suppuration is characteristic in contrast to infection due to staphylococci. Infection may also result in chronic dermatitis and disseminate to cause sepsis or endocarditis. Untreated local infection will usually abate within 3 weeks whereas therapy with oral penicillin produces a much more rapid resolution.

Erythema nodosum

These red tender nodular lesions, usually on the pretibial surface of the legs, represent a delayed hypersensitivity skin reaction. The most common precipitating factor is medication, in particular, contraceptive pills taken by adolescents. However, infectious diseases are also often incriminated, particularly GABHS (Figure 198), tuberculosis, sarcoidosis, cat-scratch disease and coccidioidomycosis (Figure 199).

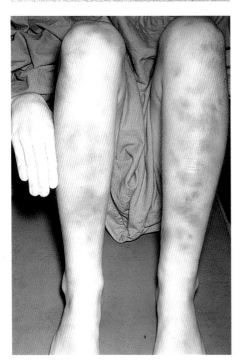

Figure 198

The nodular lesions of erythema nodosum have indistinct borders and persist for 2–6 weeks.

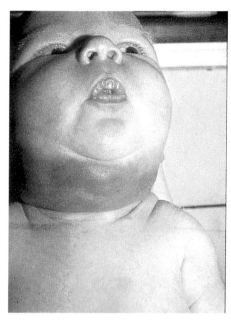

Figure 200

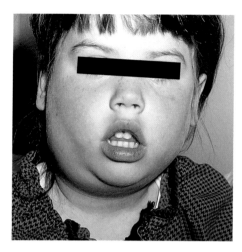

Figure 202

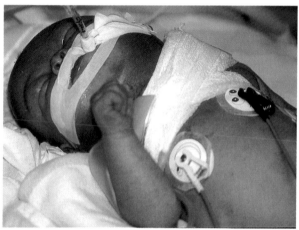

Figure 201

Ludwig's angina

An extensive, rapidly progressive cellulitis of the floor of the mouth may result in sepsis and/or airway obstruction (Figure 200). The causative pathogens, in order of frequency, are *Staphylococcus aureus*, *Streptococcus pneumoniae*, *Haemophilus influenzae*, *Escherichia coli*, *Pseudomonas* species, *Moraxella catarrhalis*, fusiform bacilli and anaerobic streptococci.

Treatment includes maintenance of the airway, usually with endotracheal intubation (Figure 201), intravenous antibiotics and surgical drainage if fluctuation is present.

Mumps

Parotitis is rarely seen in the USA and other developed countries, a result of the routine administration of measles–mumps–rubella (MMR) vaccine which began in the early 1970s.

Mumps is characterized by a gradual enlargement of one parotid gland over the course of 1–3 days (Figure 202). This may be followed by involvement of the opposite parotid gland in 25–35% of cases and often the submaxillary glands on the affected sides as well. Swelling of either or both parotid glands increases for several days. Although there is only mild tenderness on palpation, there may be intense parotid pain with chewing. Fever is of a low grade (< 102 °F).

Parotid swelling begins to subside after several days and resolves after 2–3 weeks. In an estimated 50% of infections, mumps is so mild as to remain undiagnosed.

Otitis externa

Retention of water within the ear may result in bacterial replication and inflammation of the external ear canal (Figure 203). Recovered pathogens are those which commonly colonize the skin and thrive in moist environments, such as *Pseudomonas aeruginosa*, *Staphylococcus aureus*, *Proteus vulgaris* and other Enterobacteriaceae.

Therapy of otitis externa is directed at eradication of probable organisms with broad-spectrum topical

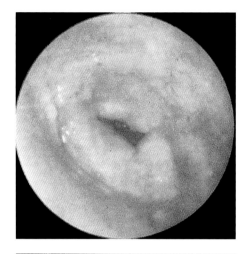

Figure 203

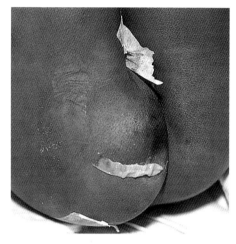

Figure 205

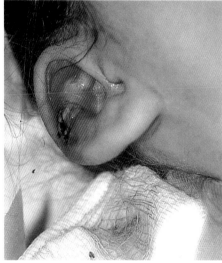

Figure 204

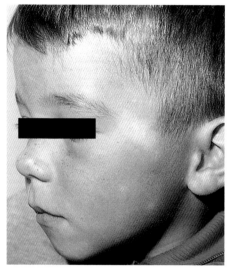

Figure 206

antibiotics, which can be accomplished with a brief 5–7-day course. Children who swim frequently or have had repeated bouts of otitis externa should instill an acidified alcohol solution into the external canals after swimming or showering.

A serious form of this infection, caused by *P. aeruginosa* (Figure 204), is seen in insulin-dependent diabetics and patients with immunodeficiency. The organism has a unique propensity for cartilage and may rapidly extend into deeper structures.

Perianal abscess

Abscesses in the perianal region (Figure 205) are almost always associated with anaerobic bacteria, although mixed infection with *Staphylococcus aureus*, *Escherichia coli*, streptococci and other coliforms is common. As with all cutaneous abscesses, incision with drainage is the most important aspect of therapy. In contrast to infection in other anatomical areas, simple drainage may be inadequate. Fistulae must be identified, opened and excised. Perianal (perirectal) abscesses therefore require surgical consultation. Antimicrobial therapy is only necessary for extensive cellulitis, systemic symptoms or an immunocompromised host.

Pityriasis alba

This common skin disorder of unknown etiology is characterized by the appearance of one or more hypopigmented patches on the face (usually the cheek; Figure 206), neck and upper trunk. The patches measure from one to several centimeters in diameter and have distinct margins; there may be fine brawny scales. The lesions are more prominent in darker-skinned subjects with recent sun exposure

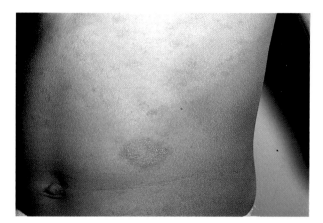

Figure 207

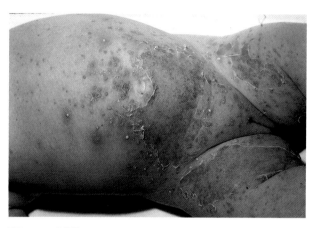

Figure 209

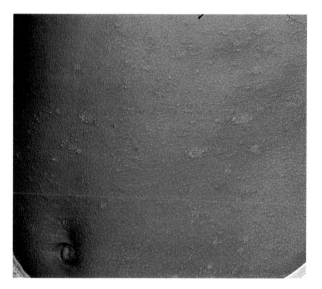

Figure 208

and tanning of the adjacent skin. The rash resolves spontaneously within several weeks.

Pityriasis rosea

The characteristic skin eruption of pityriasis rosea usually permits early clinical diagnosis. The disease is seen in school-age children and adolescents, and begins with a single skin lesion, the 'herald patch' (Figure 207). This single, round or oval, reddish-brown lesion appears on the trunk or proximal extremities, where it may resemble tinea corporis. The patch is one to several centimeters in diameter with fine scaling and elevation of the outer border, and appears several days before the generalized eruption.

Although individual skin lesions in the later rash are similar to the herald patch, such lesions are smaller, measuring from only a few millimeters to 1–3 cm in diameter, pink and oval-shaped. They may appear in one or several crops and persist for 2–12 weeks. The long axis of each plaque is usually aligned parallel to cutaneous lines of cleavage so that the overall configuration of lesions on the back resembles a Christmas tree. Most of these oval plaques have slightly raised edges with central clearing and a fine collarette of scales attached at the inner edge of the border (Figure 208). Mild pruritus is the only other manifestation. The cause of pityriasis rosea is unknown, but presumed to be of viral etiology.

Pyoderma

In pediatric patients, pyoderma refers to superficial purulent skin infections in early infancy, primarily staphylococcal disease in the newborn, which occurs in two clinical forms – pustular and bullous. The pustular form presents with a few to many skin pustules, primarily over the diaper area and trunk (Figure 209). This neonatal pyoderma is highly associated with infection due to phage group I, type 80/81 *Staphylococcus aureus*, strains that were most prevalent prior to 1970. These organisms are highly virulent, and often associated with invasive and life-threatening disease.

However, these strains have been largely replaced by exfoliatin toxin-producing strains, commonly phage group II, type 71 *S. aureus*. Although these strains are less invasive, superficial infections in

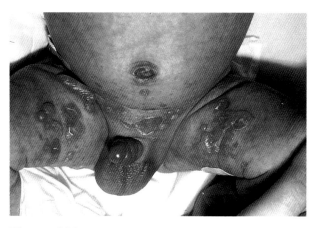

Figure 210

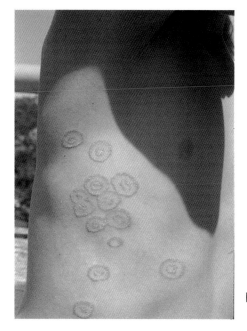

Figure 211

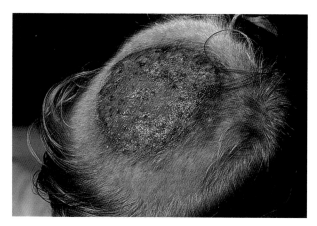

Figure 212

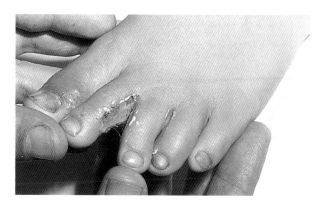

Figure 213

spreads (Figure 211). The outer edge of the lesion usually has a raised border with minute vesicles and scales. At present, the most common cause of ringworm in the USA and Europe is any of several species of *Trichophyton* including *T. tonsurans*, *T. mentagrophytes* and *T. rubrum*.

Ringworm of the scalp (tinea capitis) is manifested by circular patches of hair loss which, on close inspection, reveal individual hairs that are broken off at different levels above the scalp. There may be an intense and severe inflammatory reaction with marked boggy swelling of the area, vesicle and pustule formation, and crateriform lesions from which pus may exude, often matting the hair in a purulent crust called a kerion (Figure 212).

Other forms of skin infection due to dermatophytes that may not produce typical ringworm lesions include tinea pedis or 'athlete's foot', caused by *T. rubrum* and *Epidermophyton floccosum* (Figure 213),

newborns, who do not yet have passive immunity to their exfoliatin toxins, result in generalized erythroderma and desquamation or Ritter's disease (after the physican who first described this entity over 100 years ago). Superficial infection with these strains in newborns without passive antibodies to exfoliatin toxins results in bullous pyoderma (Figure 210).

Ringworm

Tinea corporis is an infection caused by a number of fungi (dermatophytes) that may infect the stratum corneum of glabrous skin. These infections take the form of circular lesions with expanding outer borders, often with central clearing as the infection

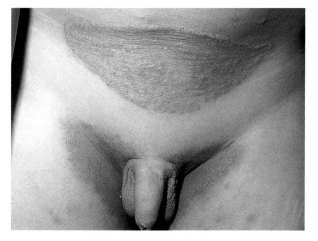

Figure 214

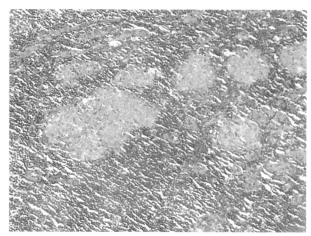

Figure 216

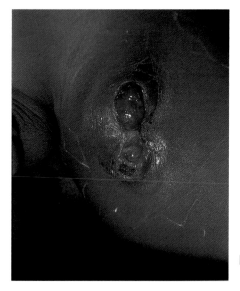

Figure 215

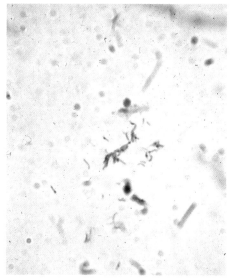

Figure 217

and *E. floccosum* infection of the groin, resulting in tinea cruris or 'jock itch' (Figure 214).

Scrofula

Although pulmonary disease is the most frequent form of tuberculosis, extrapulmonary disease following hematogenous dissemination is seen within 1 year of initial lung infection in about 25% of children < 5 years old as well as in immunosuppressed adults. Cervical lymphadenitis, termed scrofula, is the most common manifestation of disseminated tuberculosis.

This 4-year-old boy developed femoral lymphadenitis with serosanguineous discharge of 4 months' duration from which *Mycobacterium tuberculosis* was

recovered (Figure 215). His chest X-ray was normal, but the intradermal purified protein derivative (IPPD) tuberculin skin test produced a 28-mm area of induration. Biopsy of the mass revealed caseating necrosis (Figure 216), and acid-fast bacilli were identified in gastric aspirates (Figure 217). Both nodes resolved in 5 months after treatment with isoniazid and rifampin.

Non-tuberculous mycobacteria are also known to cause scrofula (Figure 218). This healthy 2-year-old had a tender parotid abscess and right submandibular adenitis for 5 weeks. Biopsy of the node revealed caseating necrosis and a culture grew *M. scrofulaceum* on Lowenstein–Jensen medium (Figure 219). A Mantoux tuberculin skin test resulted in only 6 mm of induration.

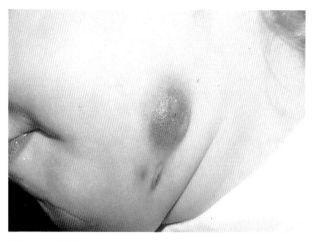

Figure 218

Isoniazid and rifampin were ineffective. Spontaneous discharge of caseous matter over several weeks was followed by incomplete healing after 6 months. Excisional surgery is the ideal therapy for non-tuberculous mycobacterial adenopathy.

Sporotrichosis

Sporothrix schenckii, a dimorphous fungus commonly isolated from soil and plants, may produce skin and subcutaneous disease in the normal host and disseminated infection in immunocompromised patients. Infection occurs in all age groups, but is most common in adult males who are likely to be exposed to contaminated soil or vegetation.

Lymphocutaneous sporotrichosis is the most common manifestation of the disease, seen in 75% of all cases. Infection follows a wound from a splinter, thorn, glass, cat bite or cat scratch contaminated with the organism.

The initial lesion is characterized by a small, firm, painless dusky-colored papule that develops at the site of trauma 1–12 weeks after inoculation, then slowly enlarges to eventually ulcerate. In children, lesions on the face and trunk are fairly common.

This child has an infection on the nose (Figure 220). Localized forms of the disorder range from scaly maculopapular lesions to verrucous and weeping ulcerations with or without satellite lesions. Itraconazole is now the treatment of choice for cutaneous sporotrichosis.

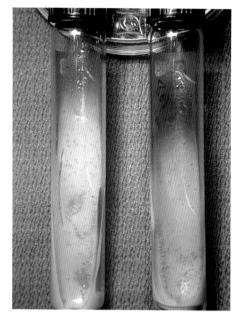

Figure 219

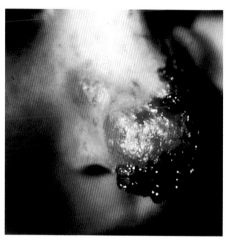

Figure 220

Swimming pool, fish-tank or Chesapeake Bay granuloma

Mycobacterium marinum is an acid-fast organism related to *M. tuberculosis* which produces chronic cutaneous lesions following injury during exposure to contaminated water. This 14-year-old presented with a 3.5-month history of a granuloma on his foot (Figure 221) which slowly developed after scraping his foot on a barnacle in the Chesapeake Bay.

A tuberculin skin test (IPPD) produced a 13-mm area of induration. Skin excisional biopsy showed non-caseating granuloma. Culture was positive for *M. marinum*. Recovery was prompt with no recurrence after 5 years.

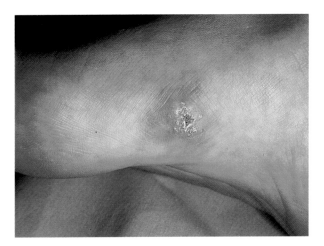

Figure 221

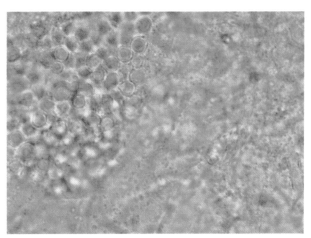

Figure 223

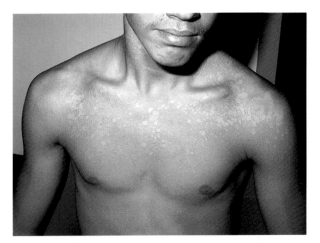

Figure 222

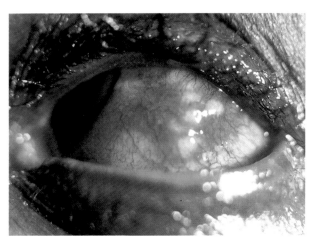

Figure 224

Tinea versicolor

This infection of the stratum corneum of the skin is caused by the dimorphic yeast *Malassezia furfur*. Round or oval hypopigmented or, less commonly, hyperpigmented lesions varying from a few millimeters to 2–3 cm in diameter occur most usually on the neck and shoulders (Figure 222). Wet-mount potassium hydroxide preparation of skin scrapings from these lesions reveal hyphae and clusters of spores (Figure 223) in a pattern often referred to as 'spaghetti and meatballs'.

Tularemia

There are six classical forms of the tick-transmitted disease caused by *Francisella tularensis*: ulceroglandular; glandular; oculoglandular, also called Parinaud's oculoglandular syndrome (Figure 224); oropharyngeal; typhoidal; and pneumonic. Pulmonary involvement is much less common in children than in adults. Regardless of disease form, the incubation period is 3–4 days; general symptoms are abrupt, consisting of fever, chills, headache and myalgia.

Treated or untreated, adenitis often progresses, thus requiring drainage for relief of symptoms (Figure 225). This needs to be carried out with caution in patients who have not completed therapy as the exudate may be infectious. Similarly, aspirated exudate should not be cultured because of risk to laboratory personnel.

Serological agglutination tests, the usual diagnostic method, are not positive until the second or third week of illness. Therefore, empirical therapy must

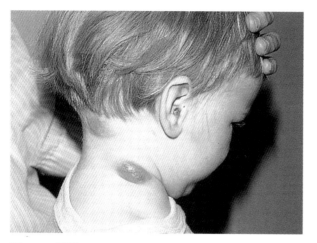

Figure 225

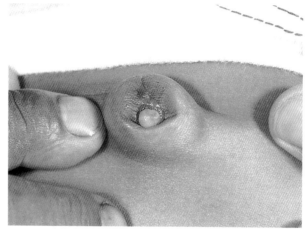

Figure 227

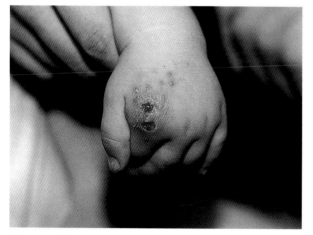

Figure 226

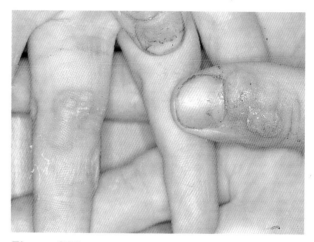

Figure 228

be considered for patients with high fever and adenitis following tick exposure in endemic regions, particularly during compatible seasons.

Disease is occasionally transmitted from the bite of an infected animal, as was the case in this 16-month-old child bitten by a pet squirrel (Figure 226). Three days following the bite, she developed cellulitis and painful axillary adenitis.

Umbilical granuloma

Pyogenic granuloma at the base of the umbilicus are commonly seen in neonates during the first few weeks of life. The lesions are round or oval, reddish-brown, smooth, firm and moist, varying in diameter from 2–3 mm to 1.0 cm or more (Figure 227). They are often pedunculated and tend to

bleed with minor trauma. Histologically, they are composed of granulomatous tissue with neovascular proliferation.

Warts (verrucae)

Human papillomavirus (HPV)-induced intraepidermal tumors are some of the most common skin disorders seen in patients of all ages. There are four basic forms of verrucae caused by different types of HPV: verruca vulgaris (due to HPV types 1, 2, 4 or 7); verruca plana (due to HPV 3, 10 or 26); verruca plantaris and condylomata acuminata (due to HPV 6, 11, 16 or 18).

The common wart appears as a single or multiple papules with an irregular rough surface (Figure 228) or, in areas of trauma, as linear warts, termed the

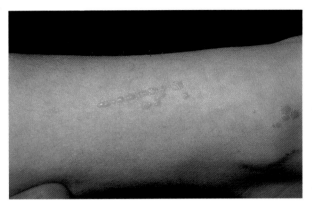

Figure 229

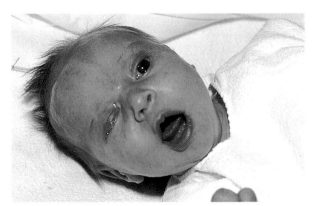

Figure 230

Koebner phenomenon (Figure 229). Lesions are usually on the extremities, but may involve other areas of the skin, including the scalp and genitalia.

Infections specific to organ systems

Bell's palsy

Also known as facial nerve paralysis, the condition is peripheral in origin. Occasionally, it is secondary to otitis media presumably as a result of extension of inflammation to cranial nerve VII as it courses through the bony canal.

This infant (Figure 230) has otitis media in the left ear and a left facial paralysis, identified by the inability to draw his mouth downwards while crying and to fully close his left eye. Paralysis may also follow viral infection, such as seen in this child (Figure 231) with a maculopapular rash, left facial nerve involvement, and a positive stool and throat culture for echovirus 9. Recent studies have documented the presence of herpes simplex virus, using the polymerase chain reaction (PCR), in a high percentage of facial nerve biopsies of Bell's palsy patients.

Brain abscess

Localized suppurative infection of the brain usually occurs by direct extension from sinus or mastoid disease. Historically, it was more commonly a sequela of bacterial meningitis but, nowadays, only meningitis caused by *Citrobacter diversus* in neonates commonly produces intracerebral abscesses. Other predisposing factors are congenital heart disease with right-to-left shunts and head trauma.

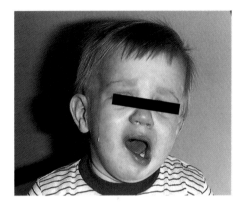

Figure 231

Clinical manifestations may be subtle, with fever, headache and vomiting being the most common. At present, computed tomography (CT) is the procedure of choice for demonstrating abscesses, as in this preoperative CT study (Figure 232), which shows a large right frontal abscess associated with maxillary and ethmoid sinus infection.

Meningoencephalitis

The majority of viral and postviral neurological diseases are benign and self-limiting, with enteroviruses causing >80% of cases in children. Some viral neurological diseases are more severe, in particular, herpes encephalitis, some equine encephalitides, and Guillain–Barré and Reye's syndromes.

Several viruses that cause meningoencephalitis appear to be clinically similar. Seasonal occurrence, and associated systemic signs and symptoms may suggest a specific viral cause. Equine encephalitis, a mosquito-borne viral disease, typically occurs during the warmer months whereas herpes encephalitis is sporadic.

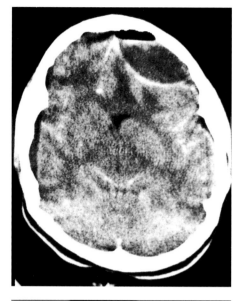

Figure 232

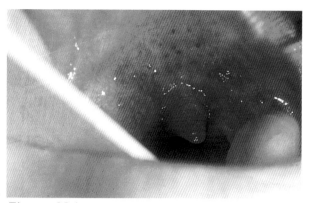

Figure 234

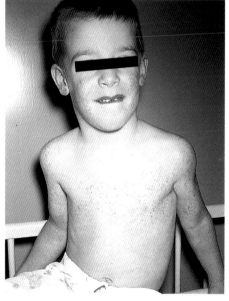

Figure 233

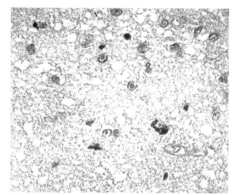

Figure 235

Cerebrospinal fluid (CSF) examination classically yields an increase in mononuclear leukocytes and red blood cells. However, as < 5% of cases have positive CSF cultures, brain biopsy for histological examination and culture is the best method for confirming the diagnosis. The site of biopsy may be determined by MRI. This brain biopsy from a 6-year-old patient shows scattered areas of cells containing cytoplasmic viral inclusions (Figure 235) indicative of herpes simplex infection.

This 4-year-old boy (Figure 233) developed persistent coryza, lethargy, headache, fever, irritability and anorexia of 3–4 days' duration. A maculopapular rash with truncal and oropharyngeal petechiae was accompanied by nuchal rigidity. Buccal pseudo-Koplik papules (Figure 234) were also observed. Echovirus 9 was isolated from pharyngeal washings.

Herpes encephalitis beyond the neonatal period usually occurs in the absence of cutaneous or other focal manifestations. Patients present with signs and symptoms of severe encephalitis such as high fever, changes in mental status, seizures and focal neurological findings.

Varicella–zoster virus has never been isolated from the CSF of an immune-competent host with encephalitis, but may be cultured from the CSF of immunosuppressed patients or identified by electron microscopy (EM), as seen in this EM from a 5-year-old (Figure 236) receiving immunosuppressive chemotherapy for leukemia who developed chickenpox and encephalitis.

Croup

Laryngotracheobronchitis (LTB) is the most common cause of acute partial upper airway obstruc-

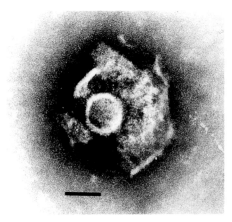

Figure 236

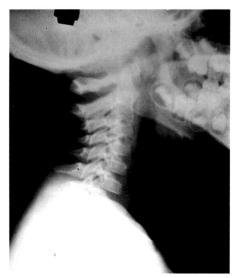

Figure 237

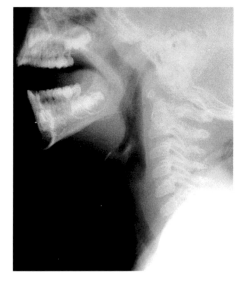

Figure 238

tion in children. The terminology used to describe this disease, and its differential diagnosis, have been confusing. LTB refers to partial airway obstruction caused by a viral infection, with erythema and edema concentrated mostly in the subglottic area. The organism responsible is usually a parainfluenza virus (types 1, 2 or 3), although other organisms may cause epidemic LTB (respiratory syncytial virus, influenza virus, rhinovirus).

The term croup is used to describe obstruction usually due to infection but, occasionally, by a foreign body or other etiology. Croup is characterized by a persistent resonant barking cough, hoarseness and stridor.

Lateral neck radiography may be helpful in differentiating the cause, whether viral, foreign body, retropharyngeal abscess or bacterial epiglottitis. These studies should be taken with the neck extended in the 'sniffing dog' position to allow optimal visualization of the trachea, larynx and supralaryngeal structures.

This normal lateral neck radiograph (Figure 237) shows the tracheal air column becoming wider and more radiolucent in the larynx. The epiglottis has the configuration of the tip of a little finger on lateral projection, the so-called little-finger sign, and the arytenoid folds are poorly visualized. The airway is patent through these structures.

In a lateral neck radiograph of a child with subglottic viral croup (Figure 238), the tracheal air column becomes narrow and less radiolucent in the larynx due to laryngeal edema, but the epiglottis is normal.

Pertussis

Whooping cough is a communicable infection of the respiratory tract characterized by repeated paroxysms of coughing. Young infants with severe disease may have numerous paroxysms terminating in cyanosis and apnea. Such episodes may be fatal if resuscitation is not provided.

This 3-month-old infant shows developing cyanosis (Figure 239) with accumulation of thick ropy airway secretions during a severe coughing paroxysm. The face of an 11-month-old child with pertussis (Figure 240), who had numerous bouts of severe coughing paroxysms daily, shows the resultant edema of the eyelids and scleral hemorrhage.

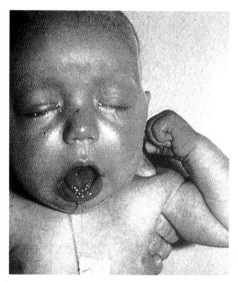

Figure 239

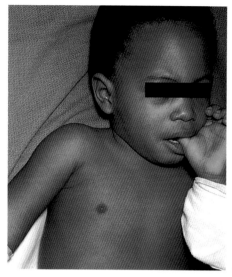

Figure 241

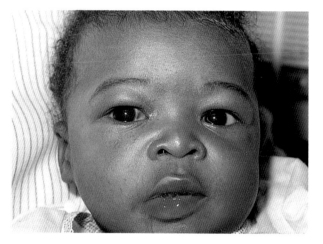

Figure 240

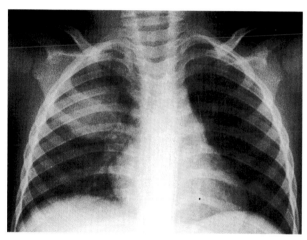

Figure 242

Pneumonia

Approximately 90% of pediatric pneumonias are caused by viral agents. Of these, 50% are attributed to respiratory syncytial virus (RSV) and 25% to parainfluenza virus types 1 and 3. A smaller number of cases are due to influenza A and B, adenovirus or rhinovirus. Three of these groups (RSV, parainfluenza virus and influenza virus) are seen almost exclusively during the winter months. Adenovirus is the common viral pathogen during the remainder of the year.

Such specific seasonal clustering of viral pneumonias suggests an increased likelihood of bacterial causes during the spring, summer and fall. Determination of the bacterial organisms causing pneumonia is primarily related to the age of the pediatric patient. Other data used to identify probable causes include associated clinical signs and symptoms, chest X-ray findings and diagnostic laboratory tests.

This 1-year-old presented with fever, cough, dyspnea, anorexia and irritability over 24 h (Figure 241). Examination revealed an acutely ill infant with tachypnea and tachycardia. Tabular breathing with dullness on percussion were noted over the right superior anterolateral chest. The white cell count was 22 000/mm^3 with 75% polymorphonuclear leukocytes and 10% band forms. Chest X-ray revealed a right upper anterior lobe pneumonia (Figure 242).

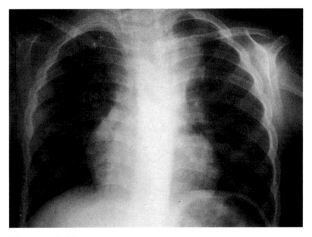

Figure 243

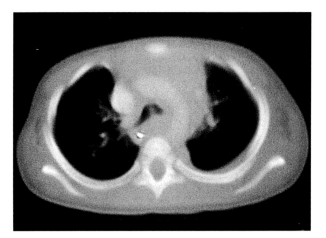

Figure 244

Blood culture grew *Klebsiella pneumoniae*. Intramuscular ampicillin for 36 h was ineffective whereas intramuscular kanamycin produced an excellent response with complete recovery 10 days after starting treatment.

Tracheal obstruction due to a mediastinal mass occurred in a 2-year-old who was hospitalized with sudden onset of stridor, dyspnea, tachypnea and fever. She had a history of persistent brassy cough and mild stridor for 5–6 weeks. The healthy mother and two siblings were tuberculin skin test-negative. The father was an expatriot of Nigeria whose health was unknown.

Chest X-ray revealed clear lung fields, but marked superior mediastinal fullness (Figure 243). CT revealed a mass compressing the trachea (Figure 244). A tuberculin skin test was positive with a 32-mm area of induration. Following endotracheal intubation, a thoracotomy revealed a 5 x 4 x 3 cm mass of matted lymph nodes.

Histological examination of an excisional biopsy showed multiple caseating granulomas containing acid-fast bacilli. *Mycobacterium tuberculosis* was cultured and was found to be susceptible to all anti-tuberculous drugs.

There was a minimal response after 18 days of treatment with intramuscular isoniazid, rifampin and streptomycin. Prednisone and dexamethasone therapy were effective, resulting in normal respiratory efforts after 5 days. Recovery was complete in 3 months, but the chest X-ray showed persistent hilar adenopathy for 5 months.

Discitis

This benign, usually self-limiting, inflammatory process or infection of the intervertebral disc space and vertebral endplate mostly affects children < 5 years of age. Responsible pathogens most commonly are *Staphylococcus aureus* or *S. epidermidis*, although cultures of the disc space are positive in < 50% of cases. Clinical manifestations include irritability, limp, refusal to sit, stand or walk and resistance to being moved.

Examination is normal except for an immobile irritable child with diffuse spinal tenderness and / or paraspinal muscle spasm. The white cell count is usually normal, but the erythrocyte sedimentation rate is often elevated. Radiography of the lumbar spine is normal during the first 2–3 weeks. However, a technetium bone scan, computed tomography or magnetic resonance imaging will reveal early intervertebral involvement.

Treatment consists of analgesics, immobilization of the spine if helpful and, in selected cases, antistaphylococcal antibiotics. The prognosis is excellent.

This 2-year-old developed severe back pain with spinal rigidity gradually over 3–4 weeks (Figure 245). He was afebrile and comfortable except when moved. There was marked spasm of the paraspinal muscles and a positive Gowers' sign. Radiography

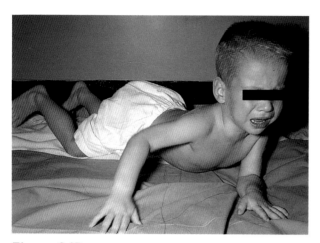

Figure 245

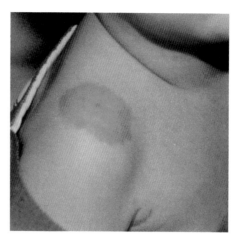

Figure 247

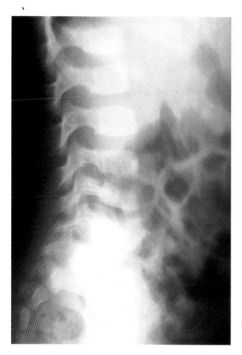

Figure 246

revealed narrowing of the L3 / L4 disc space, with irregularity of the adjacent vertebral body endplates (Figure 246).

Lyme disease

Infection caused by *Borrelia burgdorferi* begins with a characteristic rash, erythema migrans (Figure 247), at the site of a tick bite. Documentation of this rash remains the best diagnostic method as all current laboratory assays are notoriously non-specific.

By definition, the lesions are > 5 cm in diameter, often with central clearing. If untreated during the

next several weeks, patients may develop multiple similar skin lesions with periorbital edema, conjunctivitis, fever and arthralgia. Late manifestations include arthritis, carditis, facial nerve (Bell's) palsy and peripheral radiculoneuropathy.

Endemic regions in the USA are the Northeast, Midwest and California, which correlate with the distribution of the tick vectors, *Ixodes scapularis* and *Ixodes pacificus*.

Mastoiditis

This refers to infection of the posterior process of the temporal bone, almost exclusively as a consequence of prolonged middle-ear suppuration. Disease may evolve with either acute or chronic manifestations; these two presentations are distinctly different in bacterial etiology and management requirements.

The characteristic presentation is an irritable child with high fever, and retroauricular swelling and erythema which either tilts the pinna outwards and downwards or elevates the earlobe (Figure 248). This 6-month-old infant had acute mastoiditis requiring myringotomy and parenteral antibiotics.

Osteomyelitis

The pathogenesis of hematogenous osteomyelitis begins in the metaphysis of the tubular long bones adjacent to the epiphyseal growth plate. This avascular environment allows invading organisms to proliferate by avoiding influx of phagocytes, the

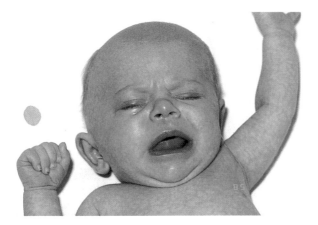

Figure 248

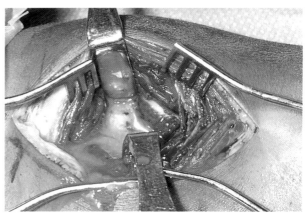

Figure 250

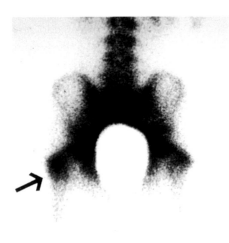

Figure 249

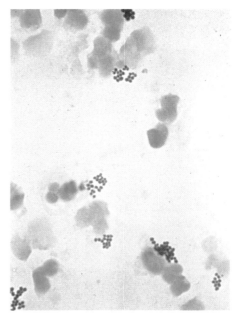

Figure 251

presence of serum antibody and complement, interaction with tissue macrophages and other host defense mechanisms. The proliferation of organisms, release of organism-related enzymes and by-products, and the fixed-volume environment contribute to the progressive bone necrosis. Signs, symptoms and pathological progression vary with the age of the patient.

This technetium-99 bone scan (Figure 249) of a child with osteomyelitis shows increased uptake in the right femur. Figure 250 shows the results of surgical drainage of the area: 220 mm of gross pus were obtained. Gram-staining of the material revealed Gram-positive cocci in clusters (Figure 251) and culture grew *Staphylococcus aureus*.

Bone changes on plain radiographs are not usually apparent until 7–14 days into the illness, as was the case in this 29-day-old infant with osteomyelitis of the proximal humerus (Figure 252) caused by group B streptococcus.

Septic arthritis

The diagnosis of septic arthritis is made earlier than in osteomyelitis due to the onset of constitutional symptoms within the first few days of infection. Patients almost always have fever, focal findings in the joint (swelling, tenderness, heat, limitation of motion) and placement of the joint in a neutral non-stressed position.

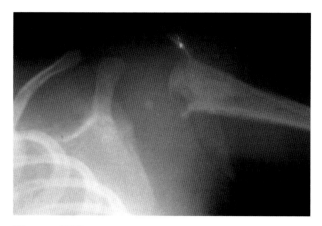

Figure 252

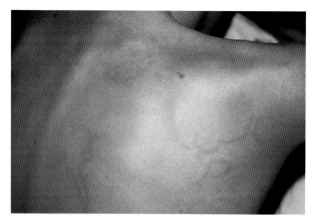

Figure 254

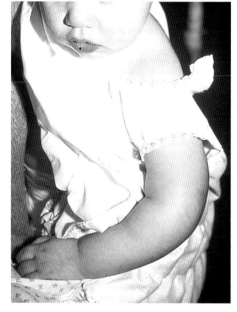

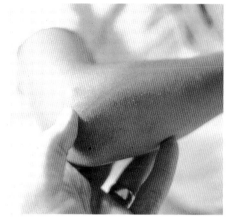

Figure 255

Figure 253

In infants, septic arthritis of the hip may have no focal findings except for positioning. Infants assume a position with the involved leg abducted, slightly flexed and externally rotated. Pain or resistance to motion should be evaluated for a possible septic hip. There is often an associated dislocation. An obvious portal of entry in septic arthritis is unusual.

This 2-year-old had fever up to 39.5 °C and a painful tender swollen left elbow for 24 h (Figure 253). Needle aspiration of the joint yielded 2 ml of straw-colored fluid. Gram-staining of the fluid revealed Gram-negative bacilli and culture grew *Haemophilus influenzae* type b.

Other infectious diseases

Rheumatic fever

There is no laboratory test or pathognomonic clinical finding to diagnose rheumatic fever. For this reason, major and minor manifestations, first described by T. Duckett Jones in 1944, are used to document the disease. Two major criteria, or one major and two minor criteria plus supporting evidence of previous group A beta-hemolytic streptococcal infection are diagnostic.

The five major criteria are carditis, migratory polyarthritis, Sydenham's chorea, erythema marginatum (Figure 254) and subcutaneous nodules (Figure 255). The minor criteria are fever, arthralgia, previous rheumatic fever or rheumatic heart disease, elevated erythrocyte sedimentation rate, positive C-reactive protein and a prolonged PR interval on electrocardiography.

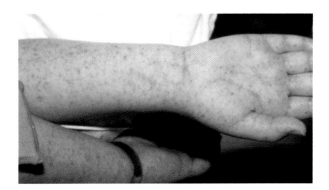

Figure 256

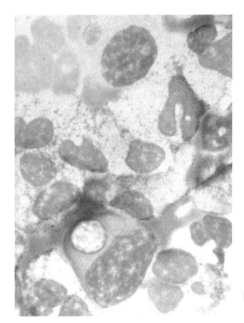

Figure 257

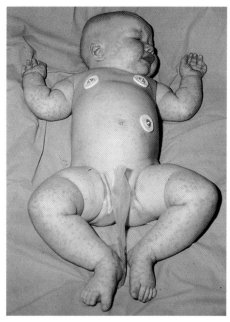

Figure 259

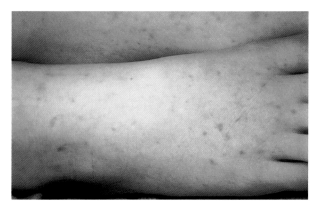

Figure 260

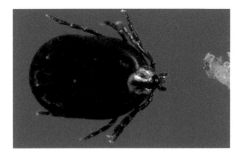

Figure 258

Ehrlichiosis

Human ehrlichiosis is a tick-borne zoonosis caused by the rickettsial organism *Ehrlichia chaffeensis*. This acute, systemic, febrile illness is clinically similar to Rocky Mountain spotted fever except that fewer than half of the patients have a rash. When present, the rash may vary from erythematous-macular to petechial (Figure 256). Other signs and symptoms, in order of frequency, are fever (95–99%), malaise (80–85%) and headache (78–84%).

Although diagnosis is usually made serologically on a four-fold or greater rise in indirect immunofluorescent titers, morulae or mulberry-like clusters of organisms may be seen in mononuclear cells in buffy-coat peripheral blood smears (Figure 257). Leukopenia and thrombocytopenia are the most consistent general laboratory abnormalities.

Rocky Mountain spotted fever (RMSF)

This is the most common rickettsial infection in the USA, and is caused by *Rickettsia rickettsii* and transmitted by the wood tick *Dermacentor andersoni* (Figure 258), the dog tick *D. variabilis* and the Lone

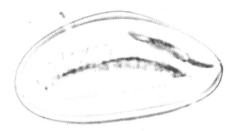

Figure 261

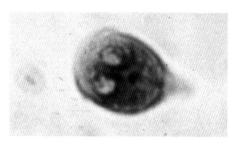

Figure 262

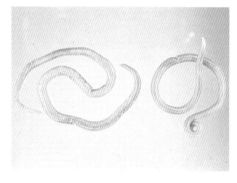

Figure 263

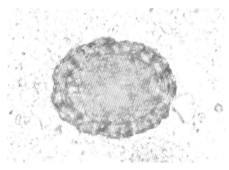

Figure 264

Star tick or *Amblyomma americanum*. Organisms replicate within the endothelial lining and smooth muscle cells of blood vessels to produce a generalized vasculitis associated with a centrifugal petechial rash and fever. Hyponatremia and thrombocytopenia are frequent laboratory features. The centrifugal distribution of the rash is evident in this 8-month-old with RMSF (Figure 259).

An 8-year-old child living in Virginia (Figure 260) developed fever up to 105 °F for 7 days, accompanied by a maculopapular exanthem for 6 days with chills, headache, photophobia and a sore throat. Oral penicillin for 4 days was ineffective. Examination was normal except for an acutely ill, lethargic child with a generalized rash and bilateral post-auricular adenopathy. Purpura and a few petechiae developed rapidly on the trunk, feet and palms. Splenomegaly was also present.

The Weil–Felix reaction was positive at a dilution of 1 : 160 for both OX-2 and OX-19 (strains of *Proteus vulgaris*), and a specific RMSF titer was positive at 1 : 8. Chloramphenicol was effective with complete recovery in 6 days.

Parasitic infections

Most parasitic diseases are now well controlled in developed countries, the result of organized efforts to improve sanitary conditions. Only pinworm (enterobiasis) and giardiasis occur frequently in pediatric practice; cases of ascariasis, amebiasis, strongyloidiasis, toxocariasis, hookworm and whipworm (trichuriasis) are only occasionally seen.

Pinworm is usually suspected in children with perianal pruritus or, rarely, vulvar pruritus. Diagnosis is confirmed by identification of *Enterobius vermicularis* eggs on clear adhesive tape (Figure 261) applied to the perianal skin when the patient first awakens in the morning. Adult nematodes which measure 2–13 mm may also be seen in the perianal region after the child has been asleep for a few hours.

Giardia lamblia is a flagellate protozoan that produces watery diarrhea accompanied by abdominal pain, which is often chronic. Trophozoites can be identified in fresh stool specimens (Figure 262), aspirated duodenal contents or on a swallowed string (Enterotest™).

Ascaris lumbricoides infestation is generally asymptomatic, although non-specific gastrointestinal symptoms, transient pneumonitis (Loeffler's syndrome) and intestinal obstruction are well described. Passage of adult nematodes, which measure 15–35 cm (Figure 263), or the presence of ova in stool (Figure 264) confirm infection. The female adult worm is larger than the male (Figure 263, left) and the male has a curved tail (Figure 263, right).

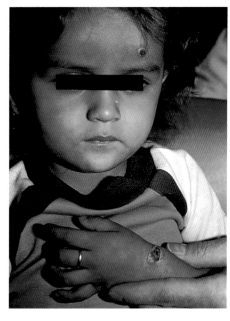

Figure 265

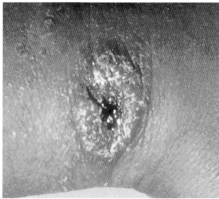

Figure 266

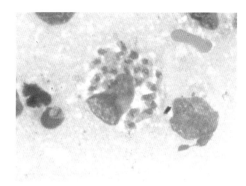

Figure 267

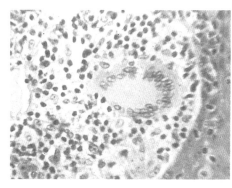

Figure 268

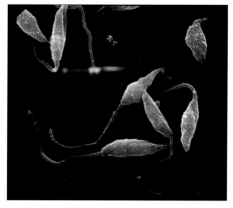

Figure 269

Leishmaniasis

Cutaneous leishmaniasis, a zoonotic infection, is caused by multiple species of the protozoan genus *Leishmania*. Subsequent to inoculation of parasites by the bite of an infected sandfly, local proliferation results in an erythematous macule or nodule that forms a shallow ulcer with raised borders.

Spontaneous resolution of lesions may take from weeks to years and usually results in residual scarring. The definitive diagnosis is established by microscopic identification of intracellular leishmanial organisms in Giemsa-stained smears or histological sections of infected tissue.

This 2-year-old boy with cutaneous leishmaniasis had granulomatous ulcerations on the forehead and

wrist which persisted and enlarged over a period of a month (Figures 265 and 266). He also had an enlarged epitrochlear node. The child had lived in Panama for 18 months and had been bitten by sandflies on numerous occasions.

Tissue aspiration of a granuloma revealed intracellular leishmanial organisms (amastigotes) on a Giemsa-stained smear (Figure 267). Biopsy of a granuloma revealed a tuberculoid reaction with lymphocytes, plasma and epitheloid cells, and Langhans' giant cells (Figure 268). Culture revealed promastigotes (Figure 269), clearly seen by electron microscopy. *Leishmania mexicana* was identified serologically by enzyme-linked immunosorbent

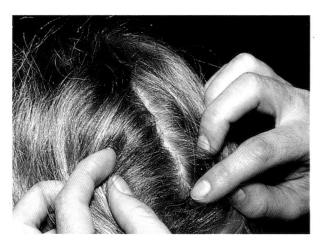

Figure 270

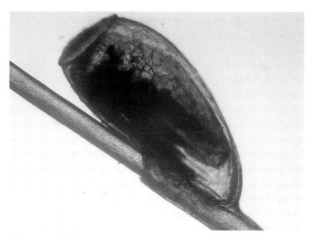

Figure 272

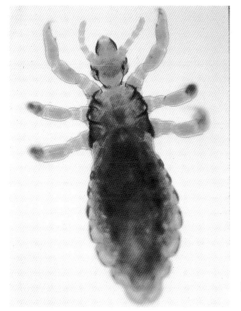

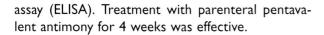

Figure 271

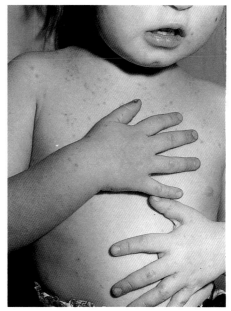

Figure 273

assay (ELISA). Treatment with parenteral pentavalent antimony for 4 weeks was effective.

Pediculosis

Lice infestation in humans may involve the head (Figure 270), where it is caused by *Pediculus humanus capitis* (Figure 271), the body (*P. humanus corporis*) or pubic hair (*Phthirus pubis*). Transmission may be direct or indirect (combs, brushes, etc.) through contact with infested subjects.

The eggs (nits) are attached to hair shafts (Figure 272), and mature and hatch within 6–10 days, leaving 'empty nits' which are not infectious. There-fore, following treatment with an appropriate pediculicide, removal of nits is unnecessary and may sometimes even be painful.

Scabies

This highly contagious, intensely pruritic dermatosis is caused by the mite *Sarcoptes scabiei* var. *hominis*, a parasite which lives out its entire lifecycle in the stratum corneum of human skin, on which it feeds. Although pruritus may be generalized, it is most intense on the hands, wrist, axilla, waist, ankles and feet, where excoriations and burrows are most often seen (Figures 273 and 274). These are the only visible signs of the disease.

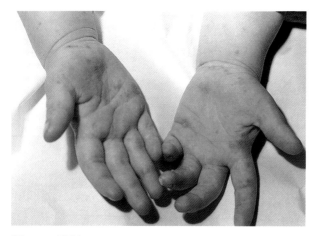

Figure 274

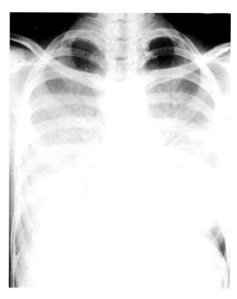

Figure 276

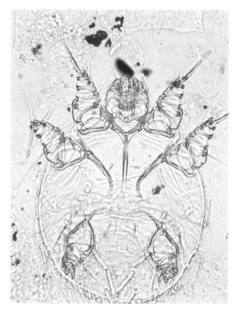

Figure 275

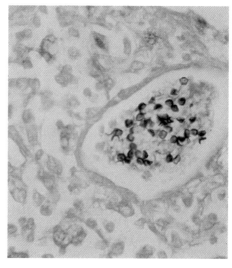

Figure 277

The female mite may be seen when curetted burrows or scrapings from the webbing between fingers are examined under the microscope in potassium hydroxide wet-mount preparations (Figure 275). In young infants, scabies lesions may be generalized and florid with papular, vesicular and pustular eruptions.

Pneumocystis carinii

Pulmonary infection with this fungus is closely associated with immunodeficiency, particularly in children with leukemia undergoing immunosuppressive chemotherapy and in those with acquired immunodeficiency syndrome (AIDS) caused by the human immunodeficiency virus (HIV).

Disease is subacute in onset, with tachypnea, acrocyanosis and cough being the predominant signs. Crackles are often subtle and unimpressive.

Chest radiography shows diffuse bilateral alveolar and interstitial disease (Figure 276). Etiological diagnosis is made by demonstration of organisms in material from bronchoalveolar lavage, endotracheal aspiration or open lung biopsy, using methenamine silver nitrate (Figure 277) or toluidine blue O stains.

Pseudomembranous and membranous colitis

Pseudomembranous colitis (PMC), an inflammation of the colon strongly associated with antibiotic use,

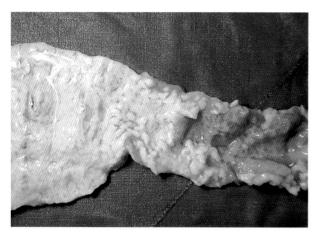

Figure 278

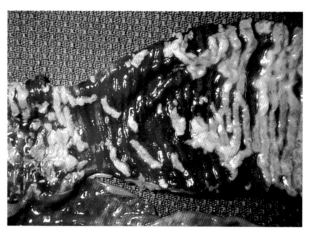

Figure 279

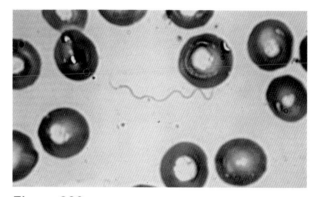

Figure 280

is caused by *Clostridium difficile* and its toxins (A and B). Although all antibiotics have been implicated, most of the cases in children have been associated with ampicillin or amoxicillin. Neither the route, dosage nor duration of treatment with the antibiotic are related to development of PMC.

The onset of diarrhea is sudden and patients may experience 10–20 stools/day, although children tend to have less severe diarrhea. Abdominal pain and tenderness may be present and may mimic an acute abdomen.

The treatment of PMC includes fluids, supportive care and discontinuation of the offending antibiotic. Approximately 25% of patients with persistent colitis require oral antimicrobial therapy. In general, metronidazole is preferable to vancomycin. The rate of relapse is 10–20%.

Peritonitis following persistent diarrhea was seen in a premature infant who had been treated with cephalothin. There was sudden abdominal distention followed by shock and death within several hours. Autopsy revealed PMC (Figure 278).

In contrast, a 4-week-old full-term infant developed severe diarrhea following removal of a meconium plug on day 2 of life. No antibiotics were given. At autopsy, extensive bronchopneumonia, peritonitis and membranous colitis (Figure 279) were found. *Staphylococcus aureus* was cultured from the lungs and peritoneal fluid. Cystic fibrosis is the most likely cause of this infant's demise.

Relapsing fever

Spirochetes of the genus *Borrelia* produce an arthropod-borne infection characterized by recurrent high fever, chills and myalgias. Cerebrospinal pleocytosis occurs in > 10% of cases. Disseminated disease may present with myocarditis, hepatic failure, cerebral edema or hemorrhage. Relapsing fever is more prevalent in the western parts of the USA, where the disease is transmitted by soft-bodied ticks of the genus *Ornithodoros*. Louse-borne disease is endemic in east and central Africa, and in the Andes in South America.

Diagnosis is usually made by identifying the corkscrew-shaped organisms on a Wright-stained peripheral blood smear (Figure 280). Serial blood smears should be obtained during febrile episodes for maximum yield. Acridine orange-staining simplifies the screening of blood smears and is more sensitive than the traditional Wright's or Giemsa stains.

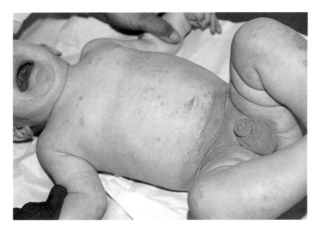

Figure 281

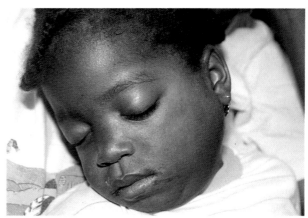

Figure 283

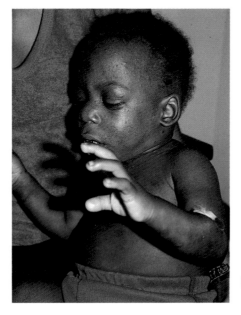

Figure 282

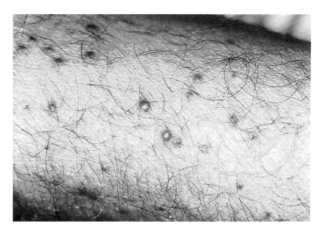

Figure 284

The immunocompromised host

Acquired immunodeficiency syndrome (AIDS)

There is a variety of initial and later clinical manifestations of human immunodeficiency virus (HIV) infection in children. Perhaps the most common manifestation is candidiasis (Figure 281), which is generally slow to resolve despite appropriate antifungal therapy. Failure to thrive with developmental delay (Figure 282) is the second most common feature, as seen in this 10-month-old infant, who weighed 6.1 kg and was unable to sit without support. Other early findings include generalized lymphadenopathy, hepatosplenomegaly, recurrent

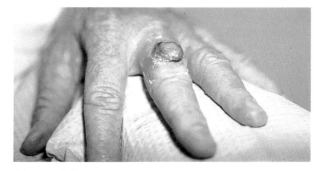

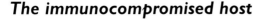

Figure 285

diarrhea, *Pneumocystis carinii* pneumonia and invasive bacterial infections.

A unique early feature is parotitis (Figure 283), which tends to be recurrent but relatively painless. HIV has been isolated from biopsies of the parotid gland in these patients, suggesting that localized viral replication with accompanying cellular infiltration is the cause of enlargement.

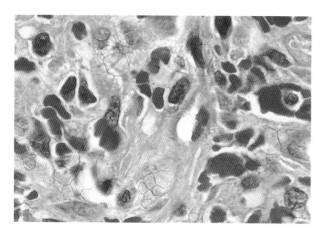

Figure 286

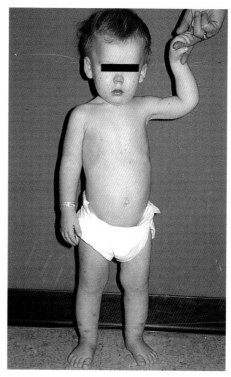

Figure 287

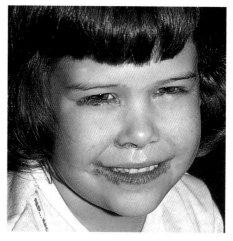

Figure 288

Bacillary angiomatosis (BA) and related visceral infection are caused by *Bartonella henselae* (which is also the etiology of cat-scratch disease), *B. quintana*, or a related organism. Disease occurs in the immunocompromised as well as occasionally in immunocompetent patients. *Bartonella* infection of the skin, liver and spleen has been recently reported in children and adults undergoing chemotherapy for cancer. The etiology is established by positive serological tests [such as an indirect fluorescent antibody (IFA) assay], positive cat-scratch antigen skin tests, presence of silvered bacilli on Warthin–Starry-staining of biopsied tissue (skin, liver, spleen, lung nodule, bone marrow) and/or positive polymerase chain reaction for *B. quintana* or *B. henselae*.

This young AIDS patient presented with multiple generalized pink and red cutaneous angiomas (Figure 284) measuring 3–5 mm in diameter. A larger 9-mm nodule had been noted on a finger (Figure 285). Biopsy of a skin lesion revealed proliferating capillaries containing large cuboidal endothelial cells with abundant cytoplasm (Figure 286), a characteristic feature of BA.

Chronic granulomatous disease (CGD)

The majority of patients with the classical X-linked form of CGD present before the second year of life with recurrent skin infections and suppurative adenitis. Pneumonia and osteomyelitis are also common. The neutrophils of these patients are able to ingest bacteria normally, but cannot kill catalase-

producing organisms such as staphylococci, *Escherichia coli*, *Serratia marcescens*, and *Salmonella* and *Candida* species. Repeated skin infections in this 2-year-old with CGD healed slowly, producing multiple scars (Figure 287). His brother had died because of staphylococcal pneumonia.

Chronic mucocutaneous candidiasis (CMC)

Inherited defects of T-cell and mononuclear phagocyte function produce a syndrome of persistent candidal infection of the mouth (Figure 288), scalp

93

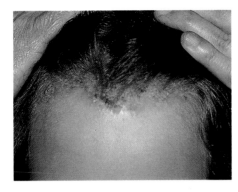

Figure 289

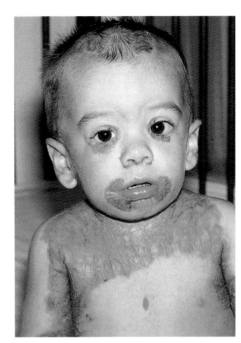

Figure 291

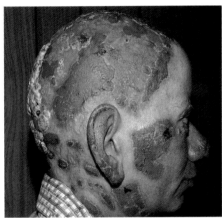

Figure 290

(Figure 289), skin (Figure 290) and nails, associated with endocrinopathies. Hypothyroidism and hypoparathyroidism are most commonly seen, but pancreatic and adrenal gland deficiencies have also been described. Endocrine gland dysfunction occurs months to years after candidiasis is apparent and may cause death if not recognized.

Newer antifungal agents such as ketoconazole or fluconazole are able to control mucocutaneous infection, as seen pre- and post-treatment (Figures 291 and 292) in a child with CMC.

Ecthyma gangrenosum

This is a rare but characteristic skin manifestation of *Pseudomonas* bacteremia, characterized by pustules or areas of cellulitis produced by septic emboli. Lesions are blackened as a consequence of hemorrhage (Figures 293) and rapidly evolve into deep ulcers with necrotic centers. Patients are severely ill with predisposing factors for *Pseudomonas* infection, such as neutropenia or following placement of central intravenous catheters. Most patients are oncology patients receiving immunosuppressive chemo-

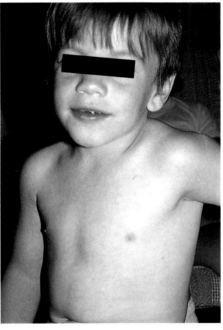

Figure 292

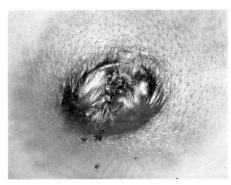

Figure 293

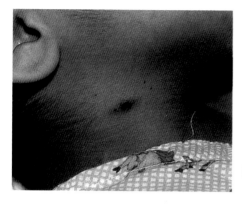

Figure 294

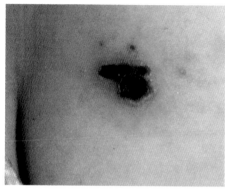

Figure 295

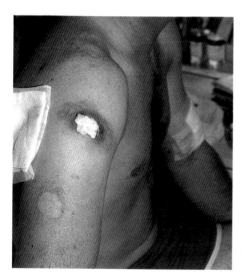

Figure 296

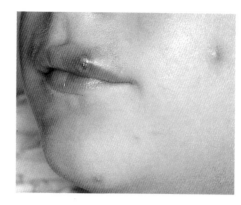

Figure 297

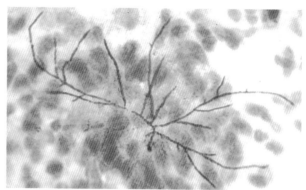

Figure 298

therapy, as in the case of this child with leukemia (Figures 294 and 295).

Hyperimmunoglobulinemia E syndrome

The combination of recurrent staphylococcal abscesses involving the skin, lungs, joints and bones associated with serum IgE levels > 1000 IU/ml, eosinophilia and atypical atopic eczema has been attributed to an imbalance of TH-1 and TH-2 lym-phocytes and is referred to as hyper IgE or Job's syndrome. This teenager (Figure 296) had deep subcutaneous abscesses caused by *Staphylococcus aureus*, a serum IgE concentration of 13 000 IU/ml and chronic eczema. His skin and lung infections began at 7 years of age. He also had a chemotactic defect of both neutrophils and monocytes.

Nocardiosis

Although all children can develop localized cuta-neous or lymphocutaneous disease caused by *Nocardia* species, an invasive infection is seen in immunocompromised patients, particularly those with chronic granulomatous disease (CGD). Infection characteristically begins in the lung with subsequent dissemination.

This 9-year-old boy with CGD had slowly progres-sive pneumonia with fever lasting 1 month, after which pustular lesions appeared on his lip and face (Figure 297). Aspiration of the lip lesion revealed beaded, branched, weakly Gram-positive rods in a classical asteroid configuration (Figure 298).

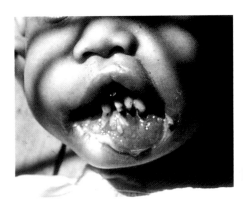

Figure 299

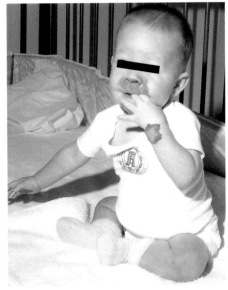

Figure 300

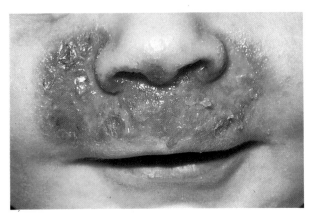

Figure 301

Noma

Also known as gangrenous stomatitis, this is a consequence of severe malnutrition leading to tissue breakdown in the oral cavity (Figure 299) and overgrowth of *Borrelia* species or other fusospirochetal

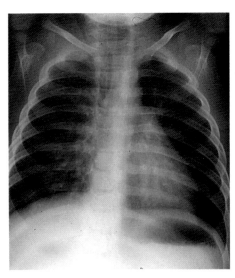

Figure 302

bacteria. This infection is only seen in developing countries where kwashiorkor and marasmus are common. Initial lesions appear as small mucous membrane ulcers that rapidly extend to the skin outside of the mouth. Treatment must include nutritional support as well as high-dose penicillin and surgical debridement.

Severe combined immunodeficiency (SCID)

The congenital absence of both T and B lymphocytes presents early in infancy with recurrent or unusual infection. Early diagnosis of this profound immune deficiency is critical, as bone marrow transplantation or enzyme replacement therapy must be provided to offer any chance of survival.

This infant (Figure 300), who was below the fifth percentile in height and weight, had two episodes of pneumonia during the first 7 months of life. He also had an unusual chronic skin infection of his upper lip (Figure 301) that was thought to be secondary to a runny nose. Chest X-ray revealed a narrow mediastinal waist indicative of an absent thymus (Figure 302). Subsequent immunological evaluation confirmed SCID. The child underwent bone marrow transplantation with his mother as donor.

Wiskott–Aldrich syndrome

This X-linked recessive disease is characterized by atopic dermatitis, thrombocytopenic purpura and

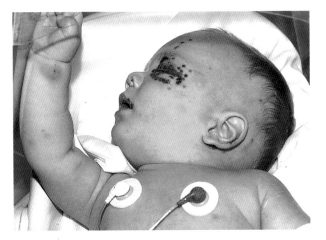

Figure 303

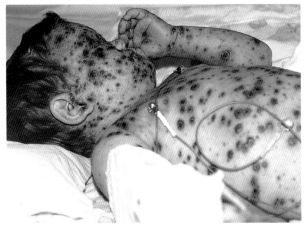

Figure 305

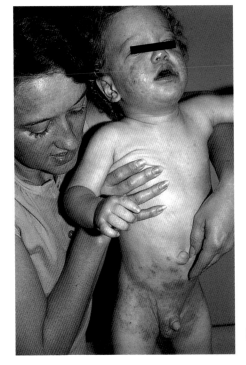

Figure 304

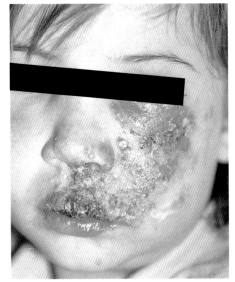

Figure 306

Zoster

an increased susceptibility to infection. The intitial presentation may be prolonged bleeding after circumcision secondary to the platelet defect, or recurrent or unusual infections later in life.

This patient initially presented at 5 months of age with ocular and periorbital herpes simplex infection (Figure 303), at which time thrombocytopenia was an incidental finding. By 18 months, he had extensive eczema (Figure 304) and, at age 3 years, severe chickenpox (Figure 305), which disseminated to the lungs and liver.

Children who are immunosuppressed have an increased risk for reactivation of varicella–zoster virus (zoster or shingles). Furthermore, in those children who have malignant disorders, infection is more likely to disseminate.

This young child with leukemia developed ophthalmic zoster (Figure 306), which was treated with intravenous acyclovir to control infection. Note that when the ophthalmic branch of the trigeminal nerve is involved, vesicles appear on the tip of the nose. In contrast, this vesicular eruption with herpes simplex (see Figure 303) does not involve the tip of the nose.

Index

A

abrasion, and cellulitis 67
abscesses 14, 15, 63
  brain 15, 78
  breast, staphylococcal infection 65
  and development of Strep-TSS 39
  hepatosplenic, in cat-scratch disease 66
  in hyperimmunoglobulinemia E syndrome 95
  perianal 63, 71
  retropharyngeal, and croup 80
  scalp 26–28
acquired immunodeficiency syndrome (AIDS)
    17, 92–93; see also immunodeficiency
  and EBV infection 42
  and Gianotti–Crosti syndrome 50
Actinomyces israelii infection, actinomycosis 63–64
acute cerebral mucormycosis 36
acute necrotizing gingivitis,
    Vincent's gingivostomatitis 59–60
adenitis
  and cellulitis, in group B streptococcus (GBS)
    infections 22–23
  preauricular, in Parinaud's oculoglandular
    syndrome 65–66
  suppurative, in chronic granulomatous disease 93
  in tularemia 76
adenopathy
  chronic, in cat-scratch disease 65, 67
  hilar, in tuberculosis with secondary pneumonia
    82

  in Kawasaki disease 44
  non-tuberculous mycobacterial 74–75
  in papulovesicular exanthematous diseases 49
  postauricular, in rubella 47
adenovirus
  in infectious mononucleosis syndrome 41
  in pneumonia 81
AIDS see acquired immunodeficiency syndrome
airway obstruction, in Hib infection 32
allergic skin rashes 40; see also drug eruptions
alopecia, hair loss 62, 73
amastigotes, in *Leishmania* infection 88
amebiasis 16
anaerobic bacteria, in perianal abscess 71
anemia 10, 22, 43
angiomatosis, bacillary, in immunodeficient patients
  93
animal bites, infection in 64–65, 75, 77
animal handling, and erysipeloid infection 68–69
anogenital molluscum contagiosum, and sexual
  abuse 52
antibiotic therapy 15; see also drug resistance
  and oral candidiasis 54
antigen-detection tests, in differential diagnosis 9
aphthae, recurrent 58
aphthous stomatitis 55, 58
aphthous ulcers, oral (herpangina) 41
Arcanobacterium hemolyticum, in pharyngitis 55
arthralgia
  in infectious mononucleosis syndrome 42

in Lyme disease 83
in maculopapular exanthematous diseases 42–43,
44, 46
in syphilis 62
arthritis
migratory polyarthritis, in rheumatic fever 85
septic 60–61, 84–85
arthritis–dermatitis syndrome, in gonococcal
infection 13, 60–61
Ascaris lumbricoides infestation, ascariasis 16, 87
ascites, in CMV infection 22
'athlete's foot', tinea pedis 73
atopic dermatitis
in HSV infection 49
in Wiskott–Aldrich syndrome 96–97
atopic eczema, in HSV infection 49
autoimmune disorders, and infection 16–17

B
bacillary angiomatosis (BA), in immunodeficient
patients 93
bacteremia, causes of 15
bacterial infections
congenital and perinatal 9–10
in conjunctivitis 21–22
differential diagnosis of 15
in pneumonia 81
and toxic shock syndrome 10–11, 14–15
bacterial meningitis *see* meningitis, bacterial
bacterial sepsis, and immunosuppression 17
Bartonella infections 14, 65–67, 69, 93
Bell's palsy, facial nerve paralysis 78, 83
blood culture, in differential diagnosis of sepsis 9
blueberry muffin skin lesions (dermal
erythropoiesis), in congenital rubella 26, 27
boils or furuncles 63
bone abnormalities, in congenital syphilis 28
bone involvement *see also* osteomyelitis
congenital rubella 26, 27
mucormycosis 36
Borrelia infections 60, 83, 91, 96
botulism, infantile 10, 30–31
brain abscess 15, 78

breast abscess, staphylococcal infection 65
bronchopneumonia, in HSV infections 24, 25
Brudzinski's sign, in bacterial meningitis 32
Bruton's X-linked hypogammaglobulinemia 16
buccal cellulitis, infective agents 67
bullous neonatal pyoderma 72
Burkitt's lymphoma, caused by EBV 42

C
cancer, immunosuppression by chemotherapy
16, 17
cancers, caused by EBV 42
Candida infection, candidiasis 16, 54, 92, 93–94
Capnocytophaga canimorsus, and animal bites 64
cardiac defects, in congenital rubella 26
cardiovascular disease
in coxsackievirus infections 49
in syphilis 62
carditis
in Kawasaki disease 44
in Lyme disease 83
myocarditis 10, 91
in rheumatic fever 85
cat-scratch disease (CSD), *Bartonella henselae*
infection 14, 65–67, 69, 93
cataracts, in congenital rubella 26
celery stalking, of the long bones, in congenital
rubella 26, 27
cellulitis 12, 15, 67–70
in bacterial meningitis 32–33
in breast abscess 65
in ecthyma gangrenosum 94
erysipelas 68
facial 22, 67, 68
cellulitis–adenitis, in group B streptococcus (GBS)
infections 22–23
central nervous system (CNS) infections 24, 25, 30,
91; *see also* encephalitis; meningitis;
neurological disorders
cephalohematoma, and scalp abscess 26–28
cerebritis, in *Toxoplasma gondii* infection 29
cerebrospinal fluid culture, in differential diagnosis
of sepsis 9, 10

cervical lymphadenitis, scrofula 74–75
cervicitis, in STD infections 61, 62
cervicofacial actinomycosis 63
chancroid, diagnosis of 13
chemotherapy
    cytolytic, and Vincent's gingivostomatitis 60
    immunosuppression by 16, 17
Chesapeake Bay granuloma 75, 76
chest radiography, in differential diagnosis 10
chickenpox, varicella infection 53–54
    disseminated, in Wiskott–Aldrich syndrome 97
    hemorrhagic, and DIC 37
    maternal 30
    and secondary erysipelas 68
child abuse see sexual abuse
chlamydial infections 13, 14, 21
chorioamnionitis, and funisitis 26
chorioretinitis 22, 29
chronic granulomatous disease 93, 95
chronic mucocutaneous candidiasis (CMC) 16,
    93–94
Citrobacter diversus, and brain abscess 78
Clostridium infections 25, 30–32, 90–91
clotting-factor deficiencies, in DIC 36
cloudy corneas, in Stevens–Johnson syndrome 59
clue cells, in vaginosis 62
CMC (chronic mucocutaneous candidiasis) 16,
    93–94
CMV see cytomegalovirus infection
CNS see central nervous system
coccidioidomycosis, and erythema nodosum 69
coliform bacteria, and conjunctivitis 22
complement deficiencies 16–17
condylomata acuminata 60, 77
condylomata lata, anogenital lesions in syphilis
    28, 29, 62
congenital heart disease, and brain abscess 78
congenital infections 9–10, 21–30
conjunctival infection, and Staph-TSS 37
conjunctivitis
    chlamydial 13
    in erythema multiforme 12
    in Kawasaki disease 44
    in Lyme disease 83
    in Parinaud's oculoglandular syndrome 65–66
    perinatal 21–22
constipation, in C. botulinum infection 30
contraceptive pills, and erythema nodosum 69
coronary aneurysm, in Kawasaki disease 44
Corynebacterium diphtheriae, in pharyngitis 55
cough
    in croup 80
    in measles 44–45
    in pertussis 80
coxsackievirus infections 12, 41, 43, 49, 50, 56–57
cranial defects, and recurrent bacterial meningitis
    34
croup, laryngotracheobronchitis (LTB) 79–80
CSD (cat-scratch disease), Bartonella henselae
    infection 14, 65–67, 69, 93
cutaneous herpes simplex infection, herpetic
    whitlow 50–51
cyclic neutropenia 16, 54–55
cytomegalovirus (CMV) infection 10, 22, 29, 41

D
deafness, in congenital infections 26, 28
dental abnormalities, in congenital syphilis 28
dermal erythropoiesis (blueberry muffin skin
    lesions), in congenital rubella 26, 27
dermal scars, in intrauterine HSV infections 24, 25
dermatitis, chronic, and erysipeloid infection 69
dermatophytes, lesions caused by 73
dermoid cysts, oral lesions 12
desquamation
    in Kawasaki disease 44
    in maculopapular exanthematous diseases 48
    in neonatal pyoderma 72–73
    in toxic shock syndromes 38, 40
developmental delay, in AIDS patients 92
'dew-drop on a rose petal' lesion of varicella–zoster
    infection 53
DGI (disseminated gonococcal infection) 60–61
diabetes mellitus
    and acute cerebral mucormycosis 36
    insulin-dependent, and otitis externa 71

diaper dermatitis, napkin rash, herpes simplex virus infection 61

diaphragmatic hernia, in group B streptococcus (GBS) infections 23

diarrhea, in Staph-TSS 37

DIC (disseminated intravascular coagulation), purpura fulminans 36–37

discitis, staphylococcal infection in 82–83

disseminated gonococcal infection (DGI) 60–61

disseminated infection, in HSV infections 24

disseminated intravascular coagulation (DIC), purpura fulminans 36–37

Downey cells 42

drug eruptions, maculopapular rashes 11, 40–41
  conjunctivitis in 21
  erythema nodosum 69
  infectious mononucleosis syndrome similarity 41–42
  and Lyell's disease 48
  pseudomembranous colitis 90–91
  and Stevens–Johnson syndrome 58

drug resistance
  in Klebsiella pneumoniae 82
  in Rocky Mountain spotted fever 87
  S. aureus and impetigo 51

drug use (illicit), and congenital syphilis 28

'drumstick' appearance, of C. botulinum bacilli 31

dyshydrosis, vesicular lesions in 12

dysphagia, in infectious mononucleosis syndrome 42

E

ear lobe petechiae, in infectious mononucleosis syndrome 42

EBV see Epstein–Barr virus

ecchymotic rash 13, 35

echovirus infections 41, 57, 78, 79

ecthyma gangrenosum, and Pseudomonas bacteremia 94–95

eczema
  in hyperimmunoglobulinemia E syndrome 95
  in Wiskott–Aldrich syndrome 97

eczema herpeticum 12, 49–50

ehrlichiosis, Ehrlichia chaffeensis infection 86

EM see erythema multiforme

emergencies, in infectious diseases 10–11, 30–40; see also omphalitis; toxic shock

enanthems 12–13, 54–60

encephalitis
  in cat-scratch disease 66
  in HSV infections 24
  in rubella infection 46
  viral 10

endocarditis 35, 61

endocrinopathies, in chronic mucocutaneous candidiasis 94

endotoxemia, in meningococcemia 35

enteric bacilli, in omphalitis 25

Enterobacteriaceae, in otitis externa 70

Enterobius vermicularis infestation, pinworm 16, 87

enteroviral infections 11, 35, 41

environmental allergens, and conjunctivitis 21

Epidermophyton floccosum infections 73–74

epidermotropic replication of viruses, and rash production 11

epiglottitis 32, 80

epistaxis, in CMV infection 22

epithelial surfaces, infection of, in diagnosis of STDs 13

Epstein pearls, oral lesions 12

Epstein–Barr virus (EBV) infections 11, 41–42, 50, 58

equine encephalitis 78

Erysipelothrix rhusiopathiae, erysipeloid infection 68–69

erythema, in cellulitis 67

erythema infectiosum 11, 42–43

erythema marginatum, in rheumatic fever 85

erythema migrans, in Lyme disease 83

erythema multiforme (EM) disorders 11, 12, 43–44, 58–59

erythema nodosum 69

erythematous macules, in leishmaniasis 88

erythematous papules, papular acrodermatitis of childhood 50

erythematous rash, in toxic shock syndromes 38, 39

erythematous-macular rash, in ehrlichiosis 86
erythrotoxigenic GABHS infection, scarlet fever 47
Escherichia coli infection
   in bacterial meningitis 33, 34
   in chronic granulomatous disease 93
   in Ludwig's angina 70
   in necrotizing fasciitis 36
   in abscesses 26–28, 71
exanthem subitum, human herpesvirus 6 (HHV-6)
   infection 46
exanthematous rashes 11–12
exanthems
   maculopapular *see* maculopapular exanthematous
      rashes
   papulovesicular *see* papulovesicular
      exanthematous diseases
exotoxin-producing staphylococci 48–49
exudative tonsillopharyngitis 55
eye disease *see also* conjunctival infection; ocular;
   ophthalmic; orbital
   in coxsackievirus infections 49
   in herpes simplex virus infections 24
   neonatal, and maternal STD 13
   and varicella–zoster infection 30
eyelid edema, in infectious mononucleosis
   syndrome 42

F
facial cellulitis 22, 67, 68
facial paralysis 30–31, 78, 83
failure to thrive
   in AIDS patients 92
   in CMV infection 22
   in SCID syndrome 96
febrile illness, assessment of 15
'fever blisters' 57
fibrosing mucoceles 12, 58
'fifth disease', erythema infectiosum 42
fish-tank granuloma 75, 76
fixed drug eruptions 40–41
foreign body, and croup 80
Francisella tularensis infection, tularemia 55, 76–77
fungal infections 15

candidiasis 16, 92, 93–94
Pneumocystis carinii 90
ringworm 73–74
sporotrichosis 75
funisitis, and chorioamnionitis 26
furuncles or boils 63
fusiform bacillae, in Ludwig's angina 70

G
GABHS *see* streptococcal infection, group A
   beta-hemolytic
gallbladder hydrops, in Kawasaki disease 44
gangrenous stomatitis, noma 96
Gardnerella vaginalis infection, in vaginosis 62
gastrointestinal disturbance 49, 55
GBS *see* streptococcal infection, group B
genital lesions in STDs 13, 28, 29, 60, 61
geographical tongue, benign migratory glossitis
   55–56
Gianotti–Crosti syndrome 12, 50
Giardia lamblia infection, giardiasis 16, 87
gingival hyperplasia, inflammatory oral lesion 12
glaucoma, in congenital rubella 26
gonococcal disease 13, 17, 60–61
Gower's sign, in discitis 82
granuloma 75, 76, 88, 93
group A beta-hemolytic streptococcal infection
   see streptococcal infection, group A
   beta-hemolytic
group B streptococci *see* streptococcal infection,
   group B
Guillain–Barré syndrome 10, 78
gummatous disease, in syphilis 62

H
Haemophilus ducreyi, diagnosis of 13
Haemophilus influenzae infection 33, 67, 70
Haemophilus influenzae type b (Hib) infection 10,
   14, 67, 68, 85
hair loss, alopecia 62, 73
hand–foot–mouth disease, coxsackievirus
   infection 56
hands, lesions on, in EM 43–44

heart *see* cardiac
hematological findings, in differential diagnosis 9
hepatic failure, in relapsing fever 91
hepatitis 28, 61
hepatitis B 13, 50
hepatosplenic abscesses, in cat-scratch disease 66
hepatosplenomegaly
   in CMV infection 22
   in congenital rubella 26
   and *E. coli* infection and scalp abscess 26–28
   in infectious mononucleosis syndrome 42
   in intrauterine infections 10
   in papulovesicular exanthematous diseases 49
   in TORCH infections 29
   in *Toxoplasma gondii* infection 29
herald patch, in pityriasis rosea 72
hernia, diaphragmatic, in group B streptococcus
   (GBS) infections 23
herpangina, aphthous ulcers 41, 56–57
herpes simplex virus (HSV) infection 13, 23–24
   in Bell's palsy 78
   eczema herpeticum 49–50
   genital, herpes genitalis 23–24, 51, 61
   gingivostomatitis 56, 57
   in immunodeficient hosts 17, 97
   in meningoencephalitis 78
   and scalp abscesses 26
   and Stevens–Johnson syndrome 58
   in TORCH presentation 10, 29
   whitlow 12, 50–51, 57
   in Wiskott–Aldrich syndrome 97
herpes zoster infection, shingles 53, 54
HHV-6 (human herpesvirus 6), roseola infantum 46
Hib *see Haemophilus influenzae* type B infection
HIV *see* human immunodeficiency virus
Hodgkin's disease, caused by EBV 42
hookworm 16
HSV *see* herpes simplex virus
human herpesvirus 6 (HHV-6), roseola infantum
   46
human immunodeficiency virus (HIV) 92–93
   in infectious mononucleosis syndrome 41–42
   and *Pneumocystis carinii* pneumonia 15

sexually transmitted 13, 14
human papillomavirus (HPV) infection 60, 77–78
hydrocephalus, in *Toxoplasma gondii* infection 29
hydrops 28, 44
hyperimmunoglobulinemia E syndrome,
   staphylococcal infection 95
hypersensitivity syndrome, erythema multiforme
   minor 43
hypogammaglobulinemia syndromes 16
hypoparathyroidism, in chronic mucocutaneous
   candidiasis 94
hypopigmentation, in pityriasis alba 71
hypothyroidism, in chronic mucocutaneous
   candidiasis 94

I

IgA deficiency (selective) 16
immune system, neonatal immaturity of 9, 14
immunocompromised host, diseases in 16–17,
   92–97
immunodeficiency 16–17
   and acute cerebral mucormycosis 36
   and candidiasis 54, 92
   and *Capnocytophaga canimorsus* infection 65
   and lymphocutaneous sporotrichosis 75
   and maculopapular exanthematous diseases
     42, 43
   and meningoencephalitis 78
   and otitis externa 71
   and perianal abscess 71
   and *Pneumocystis carinii* 90
   and scrofula 74
   in Wiskott–Aldrich syndrome, and HSV
     dermatitis 50
impetigo, as secondary infection 12, 51, 52
inclusion blennorrhea, *C. trachomatis* as cause of
   21
infections specific to organ systems 14–15,
   78–85
infectious disease emergencies 10–11, 30–40; *see
   also* omphalitis; toxic shock syndrome
infectious mononucleosis syndrome 41–42
influenza, viral 80, 81

inguinal adenopathy, in diagnosis of STDs 13
inherited disorders, susceptibility to particular
        infections 93–94, 96–97
injury see trauma
insect bites, reaction to 52–53, 67
interstitial infiltrates, on chest X-ray, in CMV
        infection 22
intestinal nematodes 16
intracerebral calcification 22, 29
intrahepatic calcifications 22
intrauterine device, and actinomycosis 63
intrauterine growth retardation 10, 24, 25, 26
intrauterine infections see congenital infections
iris lesions, in EM 43

J
jaundice 22, 29
Job's syndrome, hyperimmunoglobulinemia E
        syndrome 95
'jock itch', tinea cruris 74
Jones' criteria, diagnosis of rheumatic fever 85

K
Kaposi's varicelliform eruption, HSV infection 49
Kawasaki disease 11, 38, 44
kerion, lesion in ringworm infection 73
Kernig's sign, in bacterial meningitis 32
Klebsiella pneumoniae, in pneumonia 82
Koebner phenomenon, and linear warts 77–78
Koplik's spots, in measles 44

L
laboratory studies, for differential diagnosis of
        infections 9
laryngotracheobronchitis (LTB), croup 79–80
Leishmania infection 88–89
leukocytosis 9, 22
LGV (lymphogranuloma venereum), diagnosis of 13
lice infestation, pediculosis 89
lichenoid lesions 12, 50
linear warts, Koebner phenomenon 77–78
Listeria monocytogenes, in bacterial meningitis 33
Loeffler's syndrome, in ascariasis 87

louse-borne diseases, relapsing fever 91
LTB (laryngotracheobronchitis), croup 79–80
Ludwig's angina, oral cellulitis 70
'lumpy-bumpy jaw', in actinomycosis 63
Lyell's disease, staphylococcal scalded skin
        syndrome 48
Lyme disease, Borrelia burgdorferi infection 83
lymphadenitis
    cervical, scrofula 74–75
    chronic, in cat-scratch disease 65
    in cyclic neutropenia 55
lymphadenopathy 14, 63–78
    in AIDS 92
    in congenital rubella 26
    in herpes gingivostomatitis 56, 57
    in maculopapular exanthematous diseases
        41, 42, 46
    in syphilis 62
    in Toxoplasma gondii infection 29
lymphatic vessel involvement, in erysipelas 68
lymphocutaneous disease 75, 95
lymphogranuloma venereum (LGV), diagnosis of 13
lymphoproliferative disorders, caused by EBV 42

M
macules, definition of 11
maculopapular exanthematous rashes 11, 29,
        40–49, 62, 79, 87
malaria 16
Malassezia furfur infection, tinea versicolor 76
malignant neoplasms, oral 12
malnutrition, stomatitis 60, 96
mastoiditis 83, 84
maternal assessment, in congenital syphilis 28
maternal transmission, of STD 13; see also
        intrauterine infection
measles 11, 44–46
    and DIC 36
    and Stevens–Johnson syndrome 58–59
membranous colitis 91
meningitis
    aseptic, in coxsackievirus infection 56, 57
    bacterial 11, 15, 32–34, 78

DIC in 37
  emergency assessment of 10–11
  in gonococcal infection 61
  neonatal, incidence of 9
meningococcal infection
  and DIC 36
  and immunodeficiency 17
meningococcemia, neonatal 34–35
meningoencephalitis 78–79
menstruation, and Staph-TSS 37
microcephaly, and intrauterine infection 10, 22,
  26, 29
migratory polyarthritis, in rheumatic fever 85
Mobiluncus infection, in vaginosis 62
molluscum contagiosum 12, 51–52
Moraxella catarrhalis, in Ludwig's angina 70
morbilliform rash 11, 46
mosquito-borne diseases 16, 78
mouth *see* oral
mucocele, in salivary glands 12
mucocutaneous lesions, in syphilis 62
mucormycosis, acute cerebral 36
mulberry-like clusters, in ehrlichiosis 86
mumps, parotitis 70
Mycobacterium infections, 14, 58–59, 74, 75, 76, 82
Mycoplasma pneumoniae infection, and Stevens–
  Johnson syndrome 58–59
mycoses *see* fungal diseases
myocarditis 10, 91

N
napkin rash, diaper dermatitis, herpes simplex
  virus infection 61
nasal cavity, and acute cerebral mucormycosis 36
nasopharyngeal carcinoma, caused by EBV 42
necrotizing fasciitis 36, 37
Neisseria gonorrhoeae infection 13, 14, 21, 26, 55
Neisseria meningitidis infection 10–11, 14–15, 33,
  34–35
neonatal ophthalmia 13, 21
neonatal pyoderma 72–73
neurological disorders
  in coxsackievirus infections 49

  in herpes zoster infection 54
  neurosyphilis 28, 62
neurological disorders *see also* central nervous
  system (CNS) infections
neutropenia, in differential diagnosis 9
nevi, papular lesions in 12
Nikolsky sign, in staphylococcal scalded skin
  syndrome (SSSS) 48, 49
nits, of hair lice (pediculosis) 89
Nocardia infection, in immunodeficient hosts 95
nodular lesions, in erythema nodosum 69
noma, gangrenous stomatitis 96
non-tuberculous mycobacterial adenopathy 74–75
nuchal rigidity, in meningitis 32, 79

O
ocular changes *see also* conjunctival infection; eyes;
  ophthalmic; orbital
  in cat-scratch disease 65–67
  in Stevens–Johnson syndrome 58
oculoglandular syndromes 65–66, 76
oculomotor paralysis, in *C. botulinum* infection 31
omphalitis 25–26
opisthotonus, in neonatal tetanus 25
ophthalmia neonatorum, 13, 21
ophthalmic zoster 97
oral cellulitis, Ludwig's angina 70
oral lesions 12
  in actinomycosis 63
  aphthous stomatitis in cyclic neutropenia 55
  in candidiasis 54, 93
  in enanthems 54–60
  in herpes simplex virus infections 24
  in herpes zoster infection 53
  Koplik's spots in measles 44
  in maculopapular exanthematous diseases 43, 44
  mouth ulcers, in drug eruptions 41
  in noma 96
  in Staph-TSS 37–38
orbital cellulitis, in bacterial meningitis 33
organ systems, infections specific to 14–15, 78–85
oropharyngeal disease, in tularemia 76
osteochondritis, in congenital syphilis 28

osteomyelitis 15, 83–84
in chronic granulomatous disease 93
otitis externa 70–71
otitis media
in GBS disease 23
and secondary Bell's palsy 78
and secondary erysipelas 68

P
P. carinii pneumonia, and immunodeficiency 16, 17
palate, and acute cerebral mucormycosis 36
papillomavirus (genital warts) 13
papular acrodermatitis of childhood,
Gianotti–Crosti syndrome 50
papular rash, in cat-scratch disease 67
papular urticaria 12, 52–53
papules, definition of 11
papulosquamous rash, in syphilis 62
papulovesicular exanthematous diseases 11–12,
49–54
parainfluenza virus 50, 80, 81
parasitic infestations 16, 87–90; *see also* louse-,
mosquito- and tick-borne diseases
Parinaud's oculoglandular syndrome 65–66, 76
parotitis 70, 92
parvovirus B 19 infection, erythema infectiosum
42–43
Pasteurella multocida, and animal bites 64
Pastia's lines, in scarlet fever 47
pediculosis, lice infestation 89
pelvic actinomycosis 63–64
penile ulcer, herpes progenitalis 61
perianal abscesses 63, 71
perianal lesions in congenital syphilis 28, 29
perianal pruritus, in pinworm 87
pericarditis (purulent), bacterial, and toxic shock
11, 15
perinatal infections 9–10, 21–30
periorbital cellulitis, infective agents 67–68
periostitis, in congenital syphilis 28
pertussis, whooping cough 80
petechial rash
in ehrlichiosis 86

in gonococcal infection 60
in meningococcemia 35
oropharyngeal, in meningoencephalitis 79
in Rocky Mountain spotted fever 87
in Staph-TSS 38
in TORCH infections 29
in *Toxoplasma gondii* infection 29
pharyngitis 47, 55
PHGS (primary herpetic gingivostomatitis) 56, 57
photophobia, in measles 44
photosensitive rashes 11, 42
Phthirus pubis infestation, pubic lice 89
physical activity, and rash intensification 42
pigmentation, altered, in tinea versicolor 76
pinworm (*Enterobius vermicularis*) 16, 87
pityriasis alba 71
pityriasis rosea 72
PMC (pseudomembranous colitis), *Clostridium
difficile* infection 90–91
Pneumocystis carinii, fungal infection 15, 90, 92
pneumonia
in AIDS 92
aspiration, in *C. botulinum* infection 30
in atypical measles 46
causative agents of 81–82
chlamydial 13
in chronic granulomatous disease 93
in streptococcal infections 23, 40
and toxic shock syndrome 11, 15, 40
poliovirus infections 41
postural hypotension, in Staph-TSS 38
poxvirus infection, molluscum contagiosum 51–52
prematurity, perinatal risk factor 9
preseptal cellulitis, in bacterial meningitis 32–33
primary herpetic gingivostomatitis (PHGS) 56, 57
primary immunodeficiency 16–17
promastigotes, in *Leishmania* infection 88
proptosis, in facial cellulitis 68
prostatitis, in *Trichomonas vaginalis* infection 62
protein C, protein S deficiencies, and DIC 36
Proteus vulgaris, in otitis externa 70
pruritus
in maculopapular eruptions 40, 41, 43

perianal, in pinworm 87
in scabies 89
in sensitivity reaction to insect bites 52–53
pseudo-Koplik papules, in meningoencephalitis 79
pseudomembranous colitis (PMC), *Clostridium difficile* infection 90–91
Pseudomonas infections 70, 71, 94–95
ptosis, facial, in *C. botulinum* infection 31
pubic lice, *Phthirus pubis* infestation 89
purpura
in CMV infection 22
in drug eruptions 40
in Rocky Mountain spotted fever 87
purpura fulminans, disseminated intravascular coagulation (DIC) 36–37
purpuric lesions
in meningococcemia 35
in papular urticaria 52–53
purulent skin infection, neonatal pyoderma 72
pustular dermatitis, in infectious mononucleosis syndrome 42
pustular lesions, in gonococcal infection 60
pustular neonatal pyoderma 72
pyoderma, superficial purulent skin infections 72–73

R
rabies, management of 10
raspberry tongue, and scarlet fever 59
reactive erythema, macropapular eruptions in 11
recurrent aphthae 58
recurrent bacterial meningitis 34
recurrent herpes labialis infections 57
relapsing fever, *Borrelia* infection 91
respiratory tract disorders *see also* pneumonia
actinomycosis 64
differential diagnosis of 9–10
and maternal STD 13
in meningococcemia 35
Pneumocystis carinii infection 90
respiratory distress, in CMV infection 22
in tularemia 55, 76–77
viral infections 15, 49, 80, 81
retrovirus infections 41

Reye's syndrome 10, 78
rheumatic fever 85
rhinorrhea, in measles 44
rhinovirus 80, 81
Rhizopus infections, 36
rickettsiae, unique bacterial pathogens 15
rickettsial infections 36, 86–87
ringworm, fungal infection 73–74
Ritter's disease 48, 73
Rocky Mountain spotted fever (RMSF) 35, 86–87
roseola, maculopapular eruptions in 11
roseola infantum, human herpesvirus 6 (HHV-6) 46
rubella
congenital 26, 27
maculopapular eruptions in 11
togavirus infection 46–47
in TORCH presentation 10, 29
rubeola, measles 44–46

S
salivary glands, mucoceles in 12
Salmonella infections 26, 93
sandfly-borne infection, leishmaniasis 88
sarcoidosis, and erythema nodosum 69
Sarcoptes scabiei infestation, scabies 89–90
scalded skin syndrome, staphylococcal infection 11, 48–49
scalp, abscesses of 26–28
scarlatiniform erythroderma, in staphylococcal scalded skin syndrome (SSSS) 48–49
scarlet fever, erythrotoxigenic GABHS infection 11, 38, 47
SCID (severe combined immunodeficiency) syndrome 16, 96
scrofula, extrapulmonary tuberculosis 74–75
secondary immunodeficiency 17
secondary infection
in HSV dermatitis 50
in impetigo 51
in papulovesicular eruptions 12
in varicella lesions 54
sepsis 9, 10–11, 15, 37
septic arthritis 84–85

septicemia, and *Capnocytophaga canimorsus* infection 64

Serratia marcescens infection, in chronic granulomatous disease 93

severe combined immunodeficiency (SCID) syndrome 16, 96

sexual abuse
  and anogenital molluscum contagiosum 52
  and condylomata acuminata 60
  and sexually transmitted diseases 13–14, 61, 62

sexually transmitted diseases 13–14, 60–62

shingles, herpes zoster infection 53, 54, 97

silver nitrate application, conjunctivitis due to 21

'sixth disease', human herpesvirus 6 (HHV-6) infection 46

skin infections 11–13, 14, 24, 40–60, 63–78

'slapped cheek' red rash, in erythema infectiosum 42, 43

small for gestational age (SGA), in rubella 26, 29

smallpox (variola), papulovesicular lesions in 12

snuffles, in congenital syphilis 28, 29

soft tissue infections 14, 63–78
  necrotizing fasciitis 36, 37

spinal tenderness, in discitis 82–83

splenomegaly
  in AIDS 92
  in cat-scratch disease 66, 67
  in Rocky Mountain spotted fever 87
  in syphilis 62

sporotrichosis, *Sporothrix schenckii* fungal infection 75

SSSS (staphylococcal scalded skin syndrome) 48–49

Staph-TSS (staphylococcal toxic shock syndrome) 11, 15, 37–38, 39

staphylococcal infection
  in abscesses 26, 63, 65, 71
  and animal bites 64
  in chronic granulomatous disease 93
  in hyperimmunoglobulinemia E syndrome 95
  of the newborn, pyoderma 72–73
  in scalded skin syndrome (SSSS) 11, 48–49
  in toxic shock syndrome (Staph-TSS) 11, 15, 37–38, 39

Staphylococcus aureus infection
  and cellulitis–adenitis 23
  and conjunctivitis 22
  in discitis 82–83
  in impetigo 51
  in Ludwig's angina 70
  in necrotizing fasciitis 36
  in omphalitis 25, 26
  in osteomyelitis 84
  in otitis externa 70
  in pseudomembranous colitis 91
  in pyoderma 72–73
  in secondary infection 12

Staphylococcus epidermidis infection, in discitis 82–83

Stevens–Johnson syndrome (SJS), erythema multiforme 12, 58–59

strawberry tongue, and scarlet fever 59

Strep-TSS (streptococcal toxic shock syndrome) 39–40

streptococcal infection
  and conjunctivitis 22
  and DIC 36
  group A beta-hemolytic (GABHS)
    in abscesses 63
    in cellulitis 67
    in erysipelas 68
    and erythema nodosum 69
    in exudative tonsillopharyngitis 55
    in impetigo 51
    in necrotizing fasciitis 36, 37
    in rheumatic fever 85
    in secondary infection 12, 54
    in toxic shock syndrome 11, 15, 39–40
  group B
    in bacterial meningitis 33
    and cellulitis–adenitis 22–23
    in osteomyelitis 84
    in scalp abscesses 26, 27
    in Ludwig's angina 70
    in omphalitis 25
    in perianal abscess 71
    in toxic shock syndrome 11, 39–40

Streptococcus pneumoniae infection 10–11, 14

antibiotic resistance of 15
in bacterial meningitis 33
in Ludwig's angina 70
in periorbital cellulitis 67
strongyloidiasis 16
subcutaneous nodules, in rheumatic fever 85
submandibular adenopathy, chronic 14
submandibular cellulitis, in group B streptococcus
(GBS) infections 22
sunlight, photosensitive rashes 11, 42
suppuration, in staphylococcal infection 69
swimming pool granuloma 75, 76
Sydenham's chorea, in rheumatic fever 85
syphilis, *T. pallidum* infection 13, 14, 28–29, 62

T
target lesions, in EM 43
TEN (toxic epidermal necrolysis), in staphylococcal
scalded skin syndrome (SSSS) 48
tetanospasmin 25
tetanus, neonatal 25
thrombocytopenia
in CMV infection 22
in differential diagnosis 9
in intrauterine infection 10
in rubella infection 26, 46
thrombocytopenic purpura 36, 96–97
thrush, *Candida* infection 54
tick-borne diseases
ehrlichiosis 86
Francisella tularensis infection in tularemia 76–77
Lyme disease 83
relapsing fever 91
Rocky Mountain spotted fever (RMSF) 86–87
tinea capitis, ringworm 73
tinea corporis, ringworm 73–74
tinea cruris, 'jock itch' 74
tinea pedis, 'athlete's foot' 73
tinea versicolor, *Malassezia furfur* infection 76
togavirus infection, rubella 46–47
tongue, benign anomalies of 55–56
tonsillitis 42, 55

tonsillopharyngitis, in PHGS 57
TORCH presentation, *Toxoplasma*, rubella,
cytomegalovirus and herpes simplex infections
10, 29
torus palatinus, oral defect 12
toxic epidermal necrolysis (TEN), in staphylococcal
scalded skin syndrome (SSSS) 48
toxic granulations, in differential diagnosis 9
toxic shock syndrome 10-11, 14–15, 37–38,
39–40, 54
toxocariasis 16
toxoplasmosis 10, 29–30, 41
tracheal aspirate culture, in differential diagnosis of
sepsis 9
trauma
and aphthous stomatitis 58
and erysipeloid infection 68–69
and erythrotoxigenic GABHS infection 47
head, and brain abscess 78
and impetigo, secondary bacterial infection 51
and linear warts, the Koebner phenomenon
77–78
and lymphocutaneous sporotrichosis 75
and *Mycobacterium marinum* infection in swimming
pool granuloma 75, 76
and reactive erythema 11
and Strep-TSS 39
to the oral mucosa 12–13
trench mouth, Vincent's gingivostomatitis 59
Treponema pallidum infection, syphilis 13, 14,
28–29, 62
Trichomonas vaginalis infection 62
Trichophyton infections 73
trichuriasis (whipworm) 16
tuberculosis
and erythema nodosum 69
and secondary pneumonia 82
tuberculosis (extrapulmonary), scrofula 74–75
tularemia, *Francisella tularensis* infection 55, 76–77
typhoidal disease, in tularemia 76
Tzanck preparation, in diagnosis of herpes simplex
virus infection 61

U

ulceroglandular syndromes, in tularemia 76
ulcers
  in ecthyma gangrenosum 94
  genital, of HSV 13
  in leishmaniasis 88
umbilical granuloma 76
umbilical stump, infection of, omphalitis 25–26
urethritis, in sexually transmitted diseases 60, 62
urinary tract infection, diagnosis of 15
urine culture, in differential diagnosis of sepsis 9–10
urticaria, differentiation from EM 43

V

vaginal tampons, and Staph-TSS 37
vaginitis
  non-specific, bacterial vaginosis 62
  in *Trichomonas vaginalis* infection 62
vaginosis, bacterial, non-specific vaginitis 62
varicella infection
  chickenpox 53–54
    maternal 30
  differentiation from HSV dermatitis 50
varicella lesions, and cellulitis 67
varicella–zoster infection 10, 30, 53–54
  and DIC 36
  in immunodeficient hosts 17, 97
  in meningoencephalitis in immunodeficient host 78
  papulovesicular eruptions in 12
vascular disorders, in meningococcemia 35
vascular structures, infections in 14
vasculitis
  in meningococcemia 35
  in Rocky Mountain spotted fever 87

verruca plana 77
verruca plantaris 77
verruca vulgaris 77
verrucae (warts), human papillomavirus (HPV) infection in 77–78
verrucous lesions, in condylomata acuminata 60
vesicles, definition of 11
vesicular lesions, and varicella–zoster infection 30
Vincent's angina 59
Vincent's gingivostomatitis, acute necrotizing gingivitis 59–60
viral infections 10, 11, 15, 41–42, 78–79
vulvovaginitis, herpetic 61

W

warts (verrucae), human papillomavirus (HPV) infection 77–78
Weil-Felix reaction, in Rocky Mountain spotted fever 87
whipworm (trichuriasis) 16
white blood cell (WBC), in differential diagnosis of diseases 9
whooping cough, pertussis 80, 81
Wiskott–Aldrich syndrome 16, 50, 96–97
wounds *see* trauma

Y

Yale Observation Scale, in assessment of toxicity 10, 15
yeast, *Malassezia furfur* infection in tinea versicolor 76

Z

zoster infections, and immunodeficient hosts 97